THE COMPLETE THYROID RESET DIET COOKBOOK

AN EASY GUIDE TO ENJOY SYMPTOMS RELIEF, REVERSE HYPOTHYROIDISM, BALANCE IODINE INTAKE, ELIMINATE HYPERTHYROIDISM FOR BEGINNERS USING EASY FIBER-RICH RECIPES

CATHERINE JONES

Copyright Page

© 2023 Catherine Jones

Table of Contents

Chapter 1: INTRODUCTION

The thyroid gland is a tiny, butterfly-shaped organ that sits in front of the neck and is crucial in controlling the body's metabolism and other vital processes. It generates the hormones thyroxine (T4) and triiodothyronine (T3), which affect growth, metabolism, energy generation, and body temperature.

Since these hormones have an impact on almost every organ system, thyroid function is essential for general wellbeing. The thyroid regulates hormones in a way that keeps the body's metabolic processes in check when it is functioning at its best.

Thyroid disorders are frequently caused by imbalances in hormone production, which can result in various illnesses. For example, hypothyroidism is the condition in which the thyroid gland produces insufficient amounts of hormones. This may cause symptoms like dry skin, sensitivity to the cold, weight gain, and exhaustion. Conversely, an excess of thyroid hormones results in hyperthyroidism, which manifests as symptoms including anxiety, rapid heartbeat, weight loss, and heat sensitivity.

Thyroid nodules, which are abnormal growths inside the thyroid gland, can also develop. While the majority are benign, some can cause a goiter, or swelling of the thyroid, or interfere with hormone synthesis. These illnesses can be caused by a number of things, such as autoimmune diseases or an iodine deficit.

Thyroid-stimulating hormone (TSH), T3 and T4 levels are frequently measured by blood tests for thyroid problems diagnosis. Ultrasounds and scans are examples of imaging procedures that can be performed to evaluate the structure of the gland and find anomalies.

Thyroid problems are treated differently depending on the individual ailment. Hormone replacement therapy is the standard treatment for hypothyroidism, but drugs to lower hormone production or surgery may be necessary in extreme cases of hyperthyroidism.

It is essential for those who are suffering symptoms or want to maintain general wellness to understand thyroid health. To manage thyroid health and enhance quality of life, a balanced diet high in vital minerals such as selenium and iodine, as well as appropriate medical assistance, are necessary.

Essential Nutrients for Thyroid Support

A number of essential nutrients are essential for maintaining healthy glands and the thyroid in the best possible way. Of them, iodine is one of the most important components needed for the synthesis of thyroid hormones, specifically T3 and T4. Iodine shortage can cause hypothyroidism and goiter, two disorders that have a major impact on thyroid function.

Furthermore, the trace mineral selenium functions as an antioxidant and is necessary for the transformation of the inactive hormone T4 into the active form T3. Selenium deficiencies can impede this conversion process and throw off the thyroid hormone balance.

Additionally, copper, iron, and zinc support the health of the thyroid. Thyroid hormone synthesis is aided by zinc, whereas thyroid hormone production may be interfered with by iron deficiency. The thyroid gland's structural integrity and healthy operation are aided by copper.

Additionally, vitamins such as B12 and D are essential for thyroid function and general health. The thyroid gland has vitamin D receptors, and low levels of this nutrient may affect the production of thyroid hormones. The synthesis of red blood cells and brain function are impacted by vitamin B12, which has an indirect effect on general wellbeing and energy levels.

Maintaining appropriate iodine levels can be facilitated by eating a well-balanced diet that includes iodine-rich foods including seaweed, dairy products, iodized salt, fish, and shellfish. In a similar vein, consuming whole grains, seafood, Brazil nuts, sunflower seeds, and other sources of selenium is crucial for maintaining thyroid function.

Maintaining a healthy thyroid is mostly dependent on eating a diet high in these vital nutrients and regularly checking one's intake of iodine. Under the supervision of a healthcare provider, supplementation may be required for individuals with particular dietary issues or deficits in order to ensure healthy thyroid function.

How this cookbook can help

This cookbook functions as a thorough guide, providing doable and scrumptious foods designed to promote thyroid wellness and general wellbeing. It seeks to offer a range of tasty, nutrient-dense meals that meet the dietary requirements frequently linked to thyroid conditions.

First and foremost, this cookbook stresses the significance of eating a nutritious, well-balanced diet that is vital for thyroid function. Every recipe has been carefully designed to include components that are known to boost thyroid function, such zinc, iodine, selenium, and other essential vitamins and minerals.

It also seeks to accommodate people with different nutritional needs and preferences. This cookbook provides a selection of dishes that satisfy a variety of dietary requirements without sacrificing flavor or nutritional content, regardless of whether a person is vegetarian, vegan, gluten-free, or adheres to another specific diet plan.

The cookbook also offers helpful advice on grocery lists, cooking techniques, and meal planning. It attempts to make the process of preparing meals that support the thyroid easier by providing clear instructions that make it possible for people to easily incorporate these dishes into their everyday routines.

It also hopes to stimulate innovation in the kitchen. In addition to offering basic recipes, it promotes experimenting with thyroid-friendly ingredients so that people can discover new tastes and cooking methods that suit their nutritional needs.

Finally, the goal of this cookbook is to empower people by providing not only recipes but also deeper understanding of the larger picture of leading a healthy lifestyle. It might also provide more details on methods for managing stress, workout regimens, and other lifestyle choices that support thyroid health in general.

All things considered, this cookbook is a comprehensive tool that aims to assist people on their path to improved thyroid health by providing tasty, wholesome, and simply accessible recipes as well as lifestyle advice.

Chapter 2: ANATOMY OF THE THYROID GLAND

An important organ situated at the front of the neck, beneath the Adam's apple, the thyroid gland is responsible for controlling a wide range of physiological processes. Two lobes are joined by a small isthmus to form this butterfly-shaped endocrine gland. The thyroid plays a crucial role in homeostasis, or the preservation of the body's normal internal hormone levels, through its active hormone synthesis and secretion.

The thyroid gland is responsible for producing and secreting hormones that play a key role in controlling metabolic rate. The thyroid hormones, which include thyroxine (T_4) and triiodothyronine

(T3), affect how quickly cells in the body turn food into energy. Hormones regulate metabolic rate, which in turn affects several physiological functions like heart rate, core temperature, and cellular nutrition uptake.

An important regulator of thyroid function is thyroid-stimulating hormone (TSH), which is secreted by the pituitary gland. In response to an elevated demand for thyroid hormones, the thyroid secretes more T3 and T4 thanks to a hormone called thyroid stimulating hormone (TSH). The delicate feedback loop that aids in maintaining hormonal balance is created when increased levels of T3 and T4 decrease TSH production.

When it comes to helping kids and babies grow and develop normally, the thyroid gland is just as important. Throughout maturation of the skeletal and reproductive systems, as well as the development of the neurological system, thyroid hormones play a crucial role.

Thyroid hormone secretion of calcitonin also helps maintain normal blood calcium levels. To aid in the preservation of bone health, calcitonin lowers blood calcium levels by blocking its release from bones.

The thyroid gland is an important organ for the body's health because of its many roles in regulating many physiological processes. In order to keep the body healthy and in balance, the thyroid gland secretes hormones that influence a wide range of processes, such as metabolism, energy generation, growth, and development.

Common Thyroid Disorders

Thyroid function is regulated by the endocrine system, which includes the glands located in the neck, specifically beneath Adam's apple. A tiny isthmus connects the butterfly-shaped thyroid's two lobes. Its principal duty is to manufacture the hormones thyroxine (T4) and triiodothyronine (T3), which are essential for maintaining a healthy metabolism, producing energy, and ensuring the correct operation of different organs in the body. These hormones are secreted by the pituitary gland in response to a signal from the thyroid-stimulating hormone (TSH).

A frequent thyroid illness known as hypothyroidism is marked by an underactive thyroid, which leads to inadequate synthesis of thyroid hormones. Iodine deficiency, certain drugs, and autoimmune illnesses like Hashimoto's thyroiditis are the potential causes of hypothyroidism. Excess weight, dry skin, sensitivity to cold, and extreme tiredness are common symptoms. Usually, TSH, T_4, and T_3 levels are measured in blood tests for diagnosis. Normalizing hormone levels is the primary goal of thyroid hormone replacement therapy, which is the standard treatment.

The opposite is true in hyperthyroidism, when an overabundance of thyroid hormones is caused by an overactive thyroid gland. Hyperthyroidism is often caused by Graves' disease, an autoimmune disorder. Loss of appetite, fast heart rate, nervousness, and heat intolerance are some of the possible symptoms. Imaging investigations and blood tests (including TSH, T4, and T3 levels) are used for diagnosis. Medication to block hormone synthesis, radioactive iodine therapy, or, in extreme circumstances, thyroidectomy, are all potential treatments.

Conversely, thyroid nodules are lumps or growths that are not normally present in the thyroid gland. Some nodules may be malignant, however the majority are harmless. Thyroid nodules can have many different origins, including inflammation, a lack of iodine, or even heredity. Different nodules may cause different symptoms, or none at all. Ultrasound and fine-needle aspiration (FNA) biopsies are imaging techniques that help in diagnosis. From careful observation for benign nodules to surgical removal or radioactive iodine for malignant ones, treatment options vary according to the kind of nodule. Thyroid nodule management requires consistent monitoring and follow-up.

Risk and Prevention

An important regulator of many body processes is the butterfly-shaped thyroid gland, which is situated at the base of the neck. The thyroid is a butterfly-shaped gland that controls metabolism, growth, and development via its hormones thyroxine (T4) and triiodothyronine (T3). Its lobes are joined by a narrow isthmus. These hormones play a crucial role in regulating the body's temperature, energy levels, and general health.

Through the secretion of thyroid-stimulating hormone (TSH), the pituitary gland exerts functional control over the thyroid gland. The thyroid secretes the hormones T4 and T3 into the circulation in response to the hormone TSH. Later on, different tissues convert T4 to the highly active T3. Ensuring hormonal balance and optimal thyroid function is the complex feedback loop that involves the brain, pituitary gland, and thyroid.

Environmental and hereditary variables both play important roles in the development of thyroid problems, which are influenced by a number of risk factors. Conditions include autoimmune thyroid illnesses like Graves' disease and Hashimoto's thyroiditis, as well as benign thyroid nodules and goiters, can run in families. Thyroid function can also be affected by environmental factors, such as radiation or exposure to certain substances.

Multiple variables, including heredity, the environment, and one's way of life, must be considered in order to prevent thyroid diseases. One way to learn about such hereditary tendencies is to look at one's family tree. Thyroid function may be better monitored with the use of regular testing and doctor's visits. Reducing exposure to radiation and pollutants are examples of environmental factors that have a role in preventative initiatives.

When it comes to thyroid health, lifestyle and nutrition play a crucial role. The thyroid functions at its best when the diet is well-balanced and contains enough of iodine, selenium, and other necessary nutrients. Thyroid health is only one aspect of overall health that benefits from stress management strategies like deep breathing and getting enough sleep. It is also very important to stay away from goitrogenic foods, which can disrupt thyroid function, in excess.

Finally, the control of vital physiological processes is closely related to the thyroid gland's structure and function. Promoting thyroid health requires awareness of risk factors, implementation of preventative measures, and maintenance of a healthy lifestyle. The intricate web that supports healthy thyroid function and general wellness is supported by a combination of hereditary factors, environmental impacts, and lifestyle choices. The early diagnosis and treatment of thyroid diseases can be facilitated by proactive health measures and regular medical check-ups.

Chapter 3: THE THYROID RESET DIET

Controlling metabolic rate is the thyroid gland's principal role. Hormones produced by the thyroid regulate the metabolic rate, which in turn influences vital functions including heart rate, core temperature, and energy expenditure. For the body to stay in harmony and for all of its organs and tissues to work at their best, this control is essential.

Maintaining a healthy thyroid gland is mostly dependent on dietary factors. The synthesis of thyroid hormones relies on essential elements, including iodine and selenium. A disease known as hypothyroidism can result from a lack of iodine, which is essential for the production of thyroid hormones T3 and T4. Seafood, dairy products, iodized salt, and other seafood are good sources of iodine.

Furthermore, selenium plays a crucial role in the transformation of T4 into the more potent T3 hormone. The thyroid gland functions properly when selenium-rich foods like sunflower seeds, salmon, and Brazil nuts are consumed. Preventing thyroid-related illnesses and keeping the thyroid healthy requires a well-balanced diet that contains these micronutrients.

However, for people with thyroid diseases in particular, some foods can affect thyroid function. Overconsumption of the goitrogens found in cruciferous vegetables (e.g., broccoli, cabbage, and

Brussels sprouts) can disrupt the body's ability to produce thyroid hormone. You may lessen the goitrogenic effects of these veggies by cooking them.

In addition, the thyroid functions optimally when minerals and vitamins like zinc and vitamin D are consumed in sufficient amounts. Thyroid function is greatly impacted by vitamin D, as this vitamin contains receptors in the thyroid gland. You can keep your vitamin D levels at their best by getting enough sun exposure and eating foods that are rich in vitamin D, such fatty fish and fortified dairy products.

Ultimately, the importance of the thyroid gland to general health can only be fully grasped by delving into its structure and functioning. To keep the thyroid healthy and avoid imbalances that might cause thyroid problems, it is important to eat a balanced diet that includes iodine, selenium, zinc, and vitamin D. To get the most out of your thyroid, like with other part of your health, it's best to get expert counsel from a doctor or nurse.

Foods That Comes Highly Recommended

The goal of a thyroid reset diet is to keep hormone levels stable and the thyroid gland working at its best. The thyroid may benefit from a diet that includes nutrient-rich foods. To make thyroid hormones, you need iodine-rich foods like seaweed, dairy, and salmon. Another essential element that helps the thyroid work is selenium, which is present in Brazil nuts, sunflower seeds, and chicken.

Also, foods rich in omega-3 fatty acids, such as chia seeds, flaxseeds, and fatty fish like salmon, are part of a thyroid-friendly diet. Inflammation is detrimental to thyroid function, but these fatty acids can help alleviate it. Eating foods like nuts, seeds, and lean meats, which are rich in zinc, can help with immune system support and thyroid function.

The thyroid is frequently brought up while discussing the benefits of cruciferous vegetables, such as kale, broccoli, and Brussels sprouts. Although these veggies contain goitrogens, which might hinder iodine absorption, boiling them reduces their effect. A healthy thyroid is only one of the many benefits of a diverse and balanced diet that emphasizes whole, nutrient-dense foods.

Keep in mind that everyone's body reacts differently to different foods, so it's best to talk to a doctor or a certified nutritionist before making any major changes to your diet, particularly if you have thyroid issues.

Foods to Completely Avoid

For those who want to reset their thyroid health, here are some dietary concerns to keep in mind. In order to restore normal thyroid function and reduce inflammation, many people choose to exclude specific items from their diets as part of a thyroid reset program.

Consuming excessive amounts of cruciferous vegetables, including broccoli, cauliflower, and Brussels sprouts, might disrupt thyroid function due to the presence of chemicals called goitrogens. In a diet that is favorable to the thyroid, moderation is crucial, even though these veggies have many health advantages.

The isoflavones included in soy products may also influence the body's ability to produce and absorb thyroid hormone. People who are worried about their thyroid should cut back on soy products.

Thyroid function can be impacted by inflammation and hormonal imbalance, which can be brought about by eating too much processed foods and refined sugars. You can help your thyroid stay healthy by eating a diet full of nutrient-dense foods including fruits, vegetables, lean meats, and whole grains.

To fully grasp the thyroid gland's significance in sustaining general health, one must be familiar with its structure and function. In order to maintain good health and optimal thyroid function, it is important to eat a well-rounded diet that is favorable to the thyroid.

Chapter 4: MEAL PLANNING AND PREPARATION

The foundation of a good thyroid-focused diet is efficient and convenient meal planning and preparation, which guarantees a steady intake of nutrients that promote thyroid function.

In order to effectively prepare meals for a thyroid-conscious diet, a balanced menu comprising a range of foods high in zinc, iodine, selenium, and other vital vitamins and minerals must be created. This includes planning meals that include items such as seafood, whole grains, nuts, seeds, lean meats, and an abundance of fruits and vegetables.

Foods that support the thyroid can lose some of their nutritional content due to improper preparation techniques. Choosing to cook vegetables and meats using methods like steaming, roasting, or grilling helps retain their nutrients. A better way to prepare meals also involves reducing the usage of processed foods and bad fats.

To guarantee a steady supply of nutrients throughout the day, timing of meals is a crucial factor to take into account while meal planning. In order to sustain steady energy levels, which can improve thyroid function and general metabolic health, this entails separating meals and snacks.

Meal planning and batch cooking are useful techniques in a thyroid-focused diet. These methods make it simpler to put together wholesome meals throughout the week by preparing bigger quantities of meals or component parts in advance. This strategy reduces the temptation to choose less healthful foods out of a lack of time and helps preserve dietary consistency.

Additionally, mixing up your meal plans with a variety of foods and cuisines keeps things interesting and promotes diet compliance. To ensure that meals are thyroid-supportive and remain enjoyable, it's critical to constantly experiment with different dishes.

In general, intentionality and organization are key components of meal planning and preparation for a thyroid-focused diet. People can simplify their dietary choices to support thyroid health while keeping meals practical and enjoyable by carefully planning their meals, using thyroid-supportive items, and using effective cooking procedures.

Strategies for Efficient Meal Prep

The foundation of a good thyroid-focused diet is efficient and convenient meal planning and preparation, which guarantees a steady intake of nutrients that promote thyroid function.

In order to effectively prepare meals for a thyroid-conscious diet, a balanced menu comprising a range of foods high in zinc, iodine, selenium, A thyroid-focused diet that is successful must include effective meal prep. This will guarantee a steady intake of foods high in nutrients and make eating healthily throughout the week easier.

Start by laying out a meal plan that includes a range of foods that support the thyroid, such as zinc, iodine, selenium, and important vitamins and minerals. This plan serves as a road map to help you with your grocery shopping and cooking.

It turns out that batch cooking is a useful tactic for effective meal preparation. Set aside a certain period, like a weekend day, to cook bigger amounts of essential ingredients like grains, proteins, and chopped veggies. These ready ingredients save down on cooking time on hectic days by serving as building blocks for a variety of meals throughout the week.

Make use of adaptable components that work well in a variety of recipes. Roasted veggies, for example, go well with salads, main courses, and as fillings for wraps or sandwiches. Cooked grains, such as brown rice or quinoa, can serve as the foundation for a variety of dishes, such as dinner sides or breakfast bowls.

Purchase storage containers that make it simple to portion and retrieve prepared items. To make assembling balanced meals easier, think about utilizing mason jars or compartmentalized containers to store specific meal components.

You should think about include "one-pot" or "one-pan" meals in your meal preparation schedule. Combining several components into one cooking vessel reduces cleanup and streamlines the cooking process, all while providing a satisfying and well-rounded dinner.

To maintain freshness and make meal components easy to identify, label containers with the date of preparation and contents. This will help you stay organized. This procedure guarantees that you make effective use of prepared materials and helps to minimize food waste.

Lastly, give your meal prep procedure some leeway. While planning is important, flexibility in meal preparation helps you to accommodate shifting tastes or schedules, keeping meal prep a stress-free and sustainable part of your thyroid-focused diet.

and other vital vitamins and minerals must be created. This includes planning meals that include items such as seafood, whole grains, nuts, seeds, lean meats, and an abundance of fruits and vegetables.

Foods that support the thyroid can lose some of their nutritional content due to improper preparation techniques. Choosing to cook vegetables and meats using methods like steaming, roasting, or grilling helps retain their nutrients. A better way to prepare meals also involves reducing the usage of processed foods and bad fats.

To guarantee a steady supply of nutrients throughout the day, timing of meals is a crucial factor to take into account while meal planning. In order to sustain steady energy levels, which can improve thyroid function and general metabolic health, this entails separating meals and snacks.

Meal planning and batch cooking are useful techniques in a thyroid-focused diet. These methods make it simpler to put together wholesome meals throughout the week by preparing bigger quantities of meals or component parts in advance. This strategy reduces the temptation to choose less healthful foods out of a lack of time and helps preserve dietary consistency.

Additionally, mixing up your meal plans with a variety of foods and cuisines keeps things interesting and promotes diet compliance. To ensure that meals are thyroid-supportive and remain enjoyable, it's critical to constantly experiment with different dishes.

In general, intentionality and organization are key components of meal planning and preparation for a thyroid-focused diet. People can simplify their dietary choices to support thyroid health while keeping meals practical and enjoyable by carefully planning their meals, using thyroid-supportive items, and using effective cooking procedures.

Creating Balanced Weekly Menus

Weekly menus that are balanced and provide both diversity and practicality for meal planning are the cornerstone of a thyroid-focused diet, since they guarantee a steady intake of nutrients critical for thyroid health.

To begin with, think about eating a wide variety of foods high in zinc, iodine, selenium, and other essential vitamins and minerals for healthy thyroid function. Make sure each meal in your meal plan, which includes breakfasts, lunches, dinners, and snacks, has a combination of these nutrients.

Throughout the week, mix up your protein intake by alternating between lean meats, legumes, tofu, fish, and chicken. In addition to guaranteeing a variety of nutrients, varying protein sources adds interest to meals and helps avoid food boredom.

Your weekly menu should feature a vibrant array of fruits and vegetables. Choose a rainbow of vegetables to optimize your intake of nutrients, as different colors indicate different nutrient profiles. Berries, citrus fruits, leafy greens, and cruciferous vegetables are especially good for thyroid health.

Make sure your meals include complex carbs or whole grains, such as quinoa, brown rice, or oats. These grains enhance thyroid function and contribute to overall metabolic health by providing a consistent source of energy and vital nutrients like fiber and selenium.

Include healthy fats in your weekly menu from nuts, seeds, avocados, and olive oil. These fats supply antioxidants and omega-3 fatty acids, which promote a number of body processes, including thyroid health.

Meal balance is achieved by taking into account the distribution of macronutrients (protein, carbs, and fats) as well as portion sizes. Aim for a meal that is well-proportioned and has a combination of these ingredients to encourage fullness and a steady release of energy during the day.

Finally, be flexible and willing to change your weekly menu as needed. Since life is unpredictable, adopting a flexible approach enables you to stick to the core guidelines of a thyroid-supportive diet while accommodating schedule or preference changes.

Chapter 5: LIFESTYLE FOR THYROID WELLNESS

A comprehensive strategy for thyroid wellness takes into account lifestyle factors that can have a substantial impact on thyroid health and general well-being in addition to dietary decisions.

Frequent exercise is essential for maintaining thyroid function. Including exercise in your regimen increases energy levels, speeds up metabolism, and helps with weight management. Strength training and cardiovascular activity are both beneficial to thyroid health.

Thyroid health depends on effective stress management. Long-term stress can alter hormone levels, which may have an effect on thyroid function. Using stress-reduction strategies like yoga, meditation, deep breathing exercises, or mindfulness exercises can assist thyroid health and help control stress levels.

Sufficient sleep is essential for thyroid function and general wellness. Establish a regular sleep routine, create a relaxing environment, and prioritize relaxation before bedtime to achieve consistent and high-quality sleep.

Thyroid health benefits from minimizing exposure to endocrine-disrupting substances and environmental pollutants. To promote general wellness, try reducing exposure to chemicals, pesticides, and pollutants present in household items wherever feasible.

Thyroid health requires routine checkups and consultation with medical professionals. It is possible to diagnose thyroid issues early and treat them appropriately by monitoring thyroid hormone levels and talking with a healthcare provider about any symptoms or concerns.

Keeping up a positive social network and asking for help when you need it are crucial components of general wellbeing. Having a strong support network around you can aid in stress management and enhance mental health in general, which indirectly benefits thyroid function.

In conclusion, adopting a lifestyle that prioritizes thyroid wellness necessitates a diverse strategy. People can support thyroid health while promoting overall wellbeing by combining regular exercise, stress management strategies, getting enough sleep, reducing exposure to contaminants, receiving regular medical treatment, and cultivating a supportive social network.

Importance of Exercise

Maintaining healthy thyroid function and general health is greatly aided by exercise. Physical activity affects hormone levels, metabolism, and energy expenditure, among other thyroid health factors.

Exercise on a regular basis supports a healthy metabolism, which is directly related to thyroid function. Engaging in physical activity triggers the synthesis and secretion of thyroid hormones, enhancing metabolic efficiency and supporting weight control. This is especially important for those who have hypothyroidism because exercise helps prevent the weight gain that is frequently linked to the illness.

Additionally, exercising raises one's general energy levels. Frequent exercise helps manage feelings of weariness, stamina, and endurance—all of which are frequent in people with thyroid issues. Exercise increases energy production and reduces sensations of sluggishness by improving circulation and oxygen delivery to tissues.

Engaging in physical activity indirectly affects thyroid function while also promoting mental health. Stress, anxiety, and sadness are all known to be lowered by exercise; these factors may then impact hormone levels and thyroid function. Exercise promotes a more balanced hormonal milieu, which benefits thyroid function overall by reducing stress and elevating mood.

Furthermore, there are a variety of benefits that exercise can offer to thyroid health, such as aerobic training, strength training, and flexibility exercises. The thyroid gland is stimulated by aerobic exercises like swimming, cycling, and jogging, whereas the metabolism, muscle mass, and hormonal balance are supported by strength training.

Exercise regimens must be consistent. By promoting a consistent release of hormones and supporting metabolic processes throughout time, regular exercise helps preserve thyroid function. But, it's crucial to find a balance and refrain from overdoing it, since this might put the body under stress and perhaps have a detrimental effect on thyroid function.

All things considered, exercise is essential to thyroid health. Regular physical exercise helps people maintain a healthy metabolism, control their weight, increase their energy, elevate their mood, and support their general well-being—all of which are factors that contribute to good thyroid function.

Stress Management

It is essential to manage stress appropriately in order to maintain healthy thyroid function and general health. Long-term stress can have a substantial effect on hormone levels and may cause imbalances that influence the thyroid gland.

Stress causes the body to release cortisol and adrenaline, two hormones that can interfere with the thyroid's ability to produce and regulate thyroid hormones when they are continuously increased. This may have an impact on thyroid function, resulting in hypothyroidism or aggravating pre-existing thyroid issues.

Using stress-reduction strategies is crucial to reducing these impacts. It has been demonstrated that techniques like yoga, deep breathing, mindfulness, and meditation lower stress levels. By triggering the body's relaxation response, these methods assist in reversing the hormonal consequences of stress on the body.

Frequent exercise is another useful strategy for stress reduction. The body's natural stress relievers, endorphins, are released when you exercise, which helps to reduce tension and anxiety. Exercises like yoga, running, or even just taking a short stroll can lower stress and help thyroid function indirectly.

Stress management involves forming healthy lifestyle practices, such as getting enough sleep and eating a balanced diet. Stress can be made worse by inadequate sleep and diet, which can affect thyroid function. A nutrient-rich diet and placing a high priority on getting enough sleep are two factors that support general resilience to stress.

Additionally, setting limits and using time management techniques might help people feel less stressed. Overwhelming stress can be avoided by learning when to say no, making reasonable goals, and scheduling downtime for hobbies or leisure.

Getting help from loved ones, friends, or experts is crucial for stress management. Thyroid health can be indirectly improved by having a solid support system and obtaining counseling or treatment when necessary. These strategies can help with stress management and enhance general mental health.

People can lessen the negative effects of stress on thyroid function by embracing stress management strategies and incorporating them into their everyday lives. Effective stress management promotes a more hormonally balanced environment, which supports healthy thyroid function and general wellbeing.

Sleep for Thyroid Function

Good sleep is essential for general health and is crucial for thyroid function to work at its best. Sleep that is both restorative and adequate is necessary for the proper functioning of many hormones, including thyroid-related hormones.

The hypothalamus-pituitary-thyroid (HPT) axis, a critical system that controls the generation of thyroid hormones, is impacted by sleep, which affects the body's hormonal equilibrium. This axis can be impacted by interrupted or insufficient sleep, which may result in thyroid hormone abnormalities.

The body goes through vital processes of healing and repair when we sleep. These activities can be hampered by inadequate or poor quality sleep, which can affect hormone regulation and metabolic processes, including the production of the thyroid hormones T3 and T4. This disturbance could worsen pre-existing thyroid diseases or lead to new ones like hypothyroidism.

Regular sleep deprivation or inconsistent sleep schedules can also impact energy expenditure and metabolism, which may result in weight gain or trouble controlling weight—factors that are frequently linked to thyroid issues.

Furthermore, there is a connection between stress and sleep. Stress hormones like cortisol are released when sleep deprivation occurs, and this might affect thyroid function. Insufficient sleep can lead to elevated stress hormones, which can disrupt the HPT axis by interfering with thyroid hormone production and conversion.

Developing healthy sleeping habits is essential to maintaining thyroid function. This include sticking to a regular sleep schedule, setting up a peaceful sleeping environment, relaxing before bed, and avoiding screens or stimulating activities just before bed.

Setting aside time for 7-9 hours of sleep each night is a good way to prioritize healthy metabolism and hormonal balance, which in turn supports thyroid function. To optimize thyroid hormone regulation, sleep patterns must be consistent and restorative sleep must be ensured.

Acknowledging the significance of sleep in bolstering the body's hormonal systems, people can incorporate getting enough sleep into a comprehensive strategy to preserve good thyroid function and general health.

CHAPTER 6: EASY FIBER-RICH THYROID RESET DIET RECIPES

THYROID RESET RECIPES FOR BREAKFAST

Whipped Coffee

Ingredients

for 1 serving

- 2 tablespoons hot water (28 g)

- 2 tablespoons sugar (24 g)

- 2 tablespoons instant coffee powder (12 g)

- milk, to serve

- ice, to serve

Preparation

1. Add the hot water, sugar, and instant coffee to a bowl.

2. Either hand whisk or use an electric mixer until the mixture is fluffy and light.

3. To serve, spoon a dollop over a cup of milk with ice in it and stir.

4. Enjoy!

Fluffy Japanese Pancakes

Ingredients

for 4 servings

• 2 egg yolks

• ¼ cup sugar (50 g)

- ½ cup milk (120 mL)

- ¾ cup pancake mix (95 g)

- 4 egg whites

- butter, to serve

- syrup, to serve

- 1 cup assorted berry (175 g), to serve

Preparation

1. Mix together the egg yolks, sugar, milk, and pancake mix in a very large bowl until it is smooth with no large lumps.

2. In another large bowl, beat the egg whites with a hand mixer until stiff peaks form when lifted.

3. Carefully fold the egg whites into the pancake batter, until just incorporated, making sure not to deflate the batter.

4. Grease two 3.5-inch (9 cm) metal ring moulds and set them in the middle of a pan over the lowest heat possible.

5. Fill the moulds about ¾ of the way full with the batter, then cover the pan and cook for about 10 minutes, until the center of the pancakes are slightly jiggly.

6. Release the pancakes from the bottom of the pan with a spatula, then carefully flip them over, making sure not to spill any batter inside.

7. Cover and cook for another 5 minutes, then serve with butter, syrup, and berries!

8. Enjoy!

Cloud Eggs

Ingredients

for 2 servings

• 2 eggs

• salt, to taste

• pepper, to taste

Preparation

1. Preheat the oven to 450°F (230°C).

2. Separate the egg yolks from the egg whites. Save the yolks for later.

3. Using an electric hand whisk, whisk on a high speed until soft peaks form.

4. Fold in salt and pepper.

5. Spoon the egg whites onto a baking tray and make a well in the middle, for the yolks to go in later. Bake for 8-10 minutes.

6. Drop the yolks into the whites and bake for a further 3 minutes.

7. Serve on toast or with sides of your choice.

8. Enjoy!

Lemon-Berry Muffins

Ingredients

for 6 jumbo muffins

• 2 cups all purpose flour (250 g)

- 2 teaspoons baking powder

- ½ teaspoon baking soda

- 1 teaspoon kosher salt

- 1 stick unsalted butter, room temperature

- 1 ¼ cups granulated sugar (250 g), plus more for sprinkling

- 1 ½ teaspoons Mccormick® lemon extract

- 2 large eggs, room temperature

- ½ cup buttermilk (120 mL), room temperature

- 6 oz fresh blueberry (170 g)

Special Equipment

- muffin tin, 6 cup, jumbo

- muffin tin liner

Preparation

1. Preheat the oven to 350°F (180°C) and line a 6-cup jumbo muffin tin with liners.

2. In a large bowl, cream the butter and sugar with an electric hand mixer on medium speed until very fluffy, about 4 minutes. Add the lemon extract and continue beating for another minute. Add the eggs, 1 at a time, beating on medium speed for 30 seconds after each addition. Add the buttermilk and carefully beat to combine. The mixture will look a little grainy, but will come together once the dry **Ingredients** are added.

3. In a medium bowl, whisk together the flour, baking powder, baking soda, and salt.

4. Sift the dry **Ingredients** into the wet **Ingredients** and beat on medium-low speed to incorporate. Do not overmix.

5. Add the blueberries and carefully fold into the batter using a rubber spatula.

6. Divide the batter evenly between the prepared muffin cups, filling halfway, and sprinkle with more sugar.

7. Bake the muffins for 25-30 minutes, rotating halfway, or until light golden brown. Let the muffins cool for 5 minutes in the pan, then transfer to a wire rack to cool completely.

8. Enjoy!

Lemon Ricotta Pancakes

Ingredients

for 6 servings

- 1 pancake

- 1 cup ricotta cheese (250 g)

- 1 egg yolk

- ¾ cup milk (180 g)

- ½ teaspoon vanilla extract

- 2 tablespoons lemon zest

- 1 cup flour (125 g)

- 1 ½ teaspoons baking powder

- 1 ½ cups blueberry compote (300 g)

- 2 cups blueberry (200 g)

- ½ cup sugar (100 g)

- ½ cup water (120 mL)

• 1 tablespoon lemon juice

• 2 egg whites

• 2 tablespoons sugar

Preparation

1. In a large mixing bowl, whisk together ricotta cheese, egg yolk, milk, vanilla extract, and lemon zest. Whisk until smooth, then add flour and baking powder. Mix this until fully combined.

2. In a separate mixing bowl, beat the egg whites on high speed with an electric mixer until very white and foamy, then gradually add sugar. Continue beating on high speed until hard peaks form.

3. Gently fold ¼ of the egg whites into the lemon ricotta mixture. Gently fold in the remaining egg whites. Be careful not to deflate the eggs!

4. Butter up a nonstick pan and pour in about ¼ cup (25g) worth of batter for each pancake.

5. Cook for 2-3 minutes on each side or until golden brown on the edges.

6. In a pot or pan, cook blueberries, sugar, water, and lemon juice. Stir occasionally to prevent sticking and cook for about 8-10 minutes or until the compote reaches a thick consistency. (Compote will thicken once it cools, so to loosen it up just add a touch of hot water.)

7. Serve hot compote over stack of pancakes and dust with powdered sugar.

8. Enjoy!

Chocolate-Filled Banana Muffins

Ingredients

for 12 servings

• 2 bananas

• 1 large egg, room temperature

• ⅓ cup vegetable oil (80 mL)

• ½ cup sugar (100 g)

• ¼ cup whole milk (60 mL)

• 1 teaspoon vanilla extract

• 1 ½ cups all-purpose flour (185 g)

• 1 teaspoon baking powder

• ½ teaspoon baking soda

- ¼ teaspoon kosher salt

- ¼ cup chocolate sprinkles (50 g)

- nonstick cooking spray, for greasing pan

- ½ cup semisweet chocolate chip (90 g)

- ½ cup heavy whipping cream (120 mL), hot

Preparation

1. Preheat the oven to 300°F (150°C).

2. If your bananas aren't already very ripe, place them on a baking sheet lined with parchment paper. Bake for 15-20 minutes, until they are nearly black. Be careful to not overcook or the bananas will leak.

3. Let the bananas cool to room temperature. Increase the oven temperature to 350°F (180°C).

4. Peel the bananas, then place them in a large bowl. Mash bananas using a hand mixer or fork.

5. Add the egg, vegetable oil, sugar, milk, and vanilla. Beat until combined.

6. Sift the flour, baking powder, baking soda, and salt into the banana mixture. Beat until just combined, being careful to not overmix.

7. Use a rubber spatula to gently fold the chocolate sprinkles into the batter.

8. Grease a 12-cup muffin tin with nonstick spray. Divide the batter among the cups.

9. Bake for 20-25 minutes, until the tops are lightly browned and a toothpick inserted in the center of a muffin comes out clean.

10. Place the chocolate chips in a heatproof liquid measuring cup. Pour over the hot heavy cream. Let

sit for 1 minute, then stir until the chocolate is melted and smooth.

11. While the muffins are still warm, use the back of a wooden spoon to push down a hole into the center of each muffin. Allow to cool to room temperature.

12. Fill the muffins with the chocolate ganache.

13. Chill the muffins in the fridge for at least 1 hour, until the center has set.

14. Enjoy!

Low-Carb Bread

Ingredients

for 12 servings

- 6 egg yolks

- 6 egg whites

- 2 eggs

- 2 cups almond flour (200 g)

- ⅓ cup oil (80 g)

- 1 tablespoon baking powder

- salt, to taste

- ¼ teaspoon cream of tartar

Preparation

1. Preheat oven to 375°F (190°C).

2. Carefully separate 6 eggs, placing the yolks in a large bowl and the the whites in a medium size bowl.

3. Place the 2 whole eggs in the large bowl with the yolks and add the oil. 4. Beat together with a fork or whisk until smooth.

4. Add the almond flour, baking powder, and a pinch of salt to the egg yolk mixture. Stir the mixture with a spatula until well incorporated and set aside.

5. Add the cream of tartar to the egg whites and beat with a hand mixer until stiff peaks form.

6. Use a rubber spatula to transfer ⅓ of the whipped egg whites to the almond mixture and gently fold the batter together.

7. Add the next ⅓ of the whites to the batter and fold in until smooth.

8. Gently fold in the remaining egg whites just until the batter is smooth and no white streaks remain.

9. Line the bottom of an ungreased loaf pan with parchment paper and pour in the batter.

10. Bake for 40 minutes, until the top has set and formed a golden crust.

11. Let the loaf cool for 10 minutes before running a thin knife along the inside of the pan to release the sides of the loaf. Gently unmold the loaf from the pan and remove the parchment paper on the bottom.

12. Let the cake cool at room temperature for 1 hour before slicing.

13. Enjoy!

Blueberry Croissant Breakfast Bake

Ingredients

for 8 servings

- 1 tube crescent dough

- ¾ cup blueberry (75 g), fresh or frozen

- 8 oz cream cheese (225 g)

- ⅔ cup sugar (135 g)

- 2 eggs

- 1 teaspoon vanilla

- ¼ cup milk (60 mL)

Preparation

1. In a mixing bowl beat cream cheese, sugar, and vanilla until creamy.

2. Add eggs, and while beating slowly incorporate the milk until creamy. Set aside.

3. Preheat oven to 350°F (175°C.)

4. Using cold crescent dough, roll up crescent rolls and curve into crescent shape.

5. Place rolls in an ungreased 9x9 (23x23) pan.

6. Pour blueberries over the crescent rolls.

7. Pour cream cheese mixture over rolls and blueberries.

8. Bake at 350°F (175°C) for 35 minutes or until rolls have become golden brown.

9. Top with powdered sugar.

10. Enjoy!

Ultimate Banana Bread

Ingredients

for 1 loaf

- nonstick cooking spray, for greasing

- 1 stick unsalted butter

- 1 cup light brown sugar (200 g), plus more as needed

- 1 large egg

- 2 cups ripe banana (300 g), (about 4 large bananas)

- ½ cup full fat sour cream (120 g)

- 2 teaspoons vanilla extract

- 1 ½ cups all purpose flour (185 g)

- 1 teaspoon kosher salt

- ½ teaspoon baking soda

- 1 teaspoon ground cinnamon

- ½ cup dark chocolate chunk (85 g)

- 1 tablespoon turbinado sugar

Preparation

1. Preheat the oven to 350°F (180°C). Grease a 9 x 5-inch loaf pan with nonstick cooking spray. Line the pan with parchment paper, leaving some overhang on the long sides so it will be easy to lift out the bread, and spray again.

2. Add the butter to a medium nonstick pan over medium heat. Cook, stirring occasionally, until the butter turns amber brown and smells nutty, about 3-4 minutes. Watch carefully so the butter does not burn. Remove the pan from the heat and set aside to cool for 10–15 minutes.

3. Add cooled brown butter and brown sugar to a large bowl. Beat with an electric hand mixer on medium speed until evenly combined, about 1 minute. Add the egg and beat until light and fluffy, 3–4 minutes.

4. In a medium bowl, combine the mashed bananas, sour cream, and vanilla and mix with a rubber spatula until well combined.

5. In a separate medium bowl, whisk together the flour, salt, baking soda, and cinnamon.

6. Alternate adding the flour mixture and banana mixture to the butter mixture, starting and ending with flour and folding with a rubber spatula between each addition until just incorporated. Fold in the chocolate chunks.

7. Pour the batter into the prepared loaf pan and smooth with an offset spatula, then sprinkle the turbinado sugar on top.

8. Bake the banana bread until golden brown and a toothpick or cake tester inserted in the center comes out clean, 60–70 minutes. Set the loaf pan on a wire rack to cool for at least 1 hour, then lift out the banana bread and slice.

9. Enjoy!

Dulce De Leche Swirled Banana Bread

Ingredients

for 8 servings

• 2 cups all-purpose flour (250 g)

- 1 teaspoon baking soda

- 1 teaspoon cinnamon

- ½ teaspoon salt

- 1 ½ cups ripe banana (450 g)

- ¼ cup butter (55 g), room temperature

- ¾ cup sugar (150 g)

- 2 eggs

- ⅓ cup plain greek yogurt (95 g)

- 3 tablespoons dulce de leche

Preparation

1. Preheat the oven to 350º F (175ºC).

2. Mix flour, baking soda, cinnamon, and salt in a bowl and mix well.

3. In a separate bowl, mash the bananas.

4. Add in butter and sugar, mix until smooth.

5. Add in eggs and yogurt, mix until well-combined.

6. Add the dry **Ingredients** to the wet ingredients, mix until smooth.

7. Pour the batter into a buttered/oil-sprayed loaf pan.

8. Drop dulce de leche on top of the batter, then swirl gently into the batter with the tip of the spoon or fork.

9. Bake it for an hour and cool completely.

10. Slice and enjoy!

Strawberry Banana Crepe Cake

Ingredients

for 8 servings

- 4 large eggs

- 3 ½ cups milk (840 mL)

- ⅓ cup oil (80 mL)

- 2 teaspoons vanilla

- 3 ripe bananas, very ripe

- ½ cup sugar (100 g)

- ½ teaspoon salt

- 2 cups flour (250 g)

- ½ teaspoon unsalted butter

- 10 strawberries, stemmed, plus more, sliced for garnish

- 1 ¼ cups heavy cream (300 mL)

- 2 tablespoons powdered sugar

Preparation

1. In a food processor or blender, add the eggs, milk, oil, vanilla, bananas, sugar, salt, and flour. Blend until the batter is smooth without clumps.

2. In a medium nonstick skillet over medium heat, melt the butter and swirl so it coats the entire pan. Then pour in ¼ cup of crepe batter and tilt the pan to cover the entire bottom. Cook until the bottom surface of the crepe begins to brown and the edges are lacey, for about 3 minutes, and then flip. Repeat with the remaining crepe batter.

3. In a food processor or blender, add the strawberries and puree until smooth. Pour the strawberry puree through a sieve into a medium bowl to remove any seeds and clumps. Chill for 15 minutes until the puree is cold.

4. In a large bowl, using a whisk or hand mixer, beat the cream until thickened. Add the powdered sugar, and beat until soft peaks form. Add half of the strawberry puree, and blend with the hand mixer. Add the rest of the strawberry puree and gently fold it into the whipped cream with a spatula.

5. Dollop a bit of strawberry cream on a plate, then place the first crepe and frost with about ¼ cup of filling. Stack the remaining crepes on top of each other, with strawberry whipped cream between each layer. Spread the rest of the strawberry whipped cream on top of the last crepe.

6. Arrange slices of strawberry on top for garnish.

7. Slice and serve.

Cinnamon Roll Breakfast Muffins

Ingredients

for 12 muffins

• 6 eggs

• ½ cup milk (120 mL)

• ½ cup heavy cream (120 mL)

• 2 teaspoons vanilla extract

• 2 teaspoons cinnamon

• ½ cup sugar (100 g)

• 2 packs cinnamon roll

Preparation

1. In a medium bowl, mix eggs, milk, cream, vanilla extract, cinnamon, and sugar. Whisk together.

2. Cut each cinnamon roll into eight pieces, and stuff inside a greased muffin tin.

3. Pour batter in each tin about ¾ of the way. If you pour too much, the tin will overflow in the oven.

4. Cover the tin and refrigerate for at least 2 hours, letting the cinnamon roll absorb the mixture.

5. Bake at 350°F (175°C) for 35 minutes.

6. Remove the muffin from the tin, top with icing and serve warm.

7. Enjoy!

Sweet Potato-Pecan Cinnamon Rolls

Ingredients

for 12 servings

Rolls

- 1 cup plain unsweetened soy milk (240 mL), or other non-dairy milk

- ¼ cup vegan butter (55 g)

- 1 cup mashed sweet potato (250 g), from 1 baked medium sweet potato

- 3 cups unbleached all-purpose flour (375 g), plus more for dusting

- ¼ cup granulated sugar (50 g)

- ½ teaspoon salt

- 2 ¼ teaspoons active dry yeast, 1 packet

- ½ teaspoon grapeseed oil

Filling

- ½ cup brown sugar (110 g), or coconut sugar, or a mix of the two

- ½ tablespoon ground cinnamon

- ¾ cup toasted pecans (95 g)

- ⅓ cup vegan butter (75 g)

Sweet Potato Cream Cheese Frosting

- ½ cup vegan cream cheese (110 g)

- ½ cup confectioners sugar (80 g)

- ¼ cup mashed sweet potato (60 g), from ¼ baked medium sweet potato

• ½ teaspoon pure vanilla extract

Preparation

1. In a small saucepan, warm the soy milk and vegan butter over medium heat until the butter has melted. Do not boil it. Remove from the heat and stir in the mashed sweet potato.

2. In a large bowl, mix together the flour, granulated sugar, salt, and yeast. Pour the liquid **Ingredients** into the dry and use a wooden spoon to combine. Once it gets too difficult to stir, use your hands to combine the ingredients.

3. Flour a clean work surface and transfer the dough onto the prepared work space. Knead it until you've got a smooth dough ball. Lightly oil a large bowl. Place the dough ball in it, cover with plastic wrap or a kitchen towel, and let rise for 1 hour. The dough should double in size.

4. Make the filling: In a small bowl, combine the brown sugar and cinnamon and set aside. Chop the pecans into small pieces and set aside. In a small saucepan, melt the vegan butter and set aside.

5. Once the dough has doubled in size, preheat the oven to 375°F (190°C).

6. Press the air out of the dough, then transfer it back onto your floured work space. Roll the dough until it is about ¼-inch (6 mm) thick. You should end up with a roughly rectangular oval, about 12x16 inches (30x40 cm).

7. Brush the dough with the melted butter, sprinkle with the cinnamon-sugar mix, and then top with the chopped pecans. Fold the short side of the dough over and roll tightly until you have a log.

8. Carefully cut the log into twelve 1-inch (2 cm) slices. Grease a large skillet or a 10-inch (25 cm)

round baking dish and place the rolls in it cut-side down.

9. Bake for 25 minutes, or until they've expanded and turned slightly golden on top.

10. Meanwhile, make the frosting: Place all the **Ingredients** in a food processor or standing mixer with the whisk attachment on high and blend until creamy.

11. Remove the rolls from the oven and let cool for 5 to 10 minutes. Top with the sweet potato frosting and serve immediately. They will stay fresh for up to 2 days, but they're best eaten the day you bake them.

12. Enjoy!

Citrus Poppy Muffins With Candied Kumquats

Ingredients

for 12 servings

Candied Kumquats

- 1 cup granulated sugar (200 g)

- 1 cup water (240 mL)

- 5 kumquats, thinly sliced crosswise, seeds removed

Citrus Poppy Muffins

- nonstick cooking spray, for greasing

- 5 kumquats

- 4 tangerines

- 5 large meyer lemon

- 1 ¼ sticks unsalted butter, room temperature, plus 2 tablespoons

- 1 cup granulated sugar (200 g), divided, plus 5 tablespoons

- ½ teaspoon kosher salt

- 2 large eggs

- 2 large egg yolks

- 1 ¾ cups all purpose flour (215 g)

- 2 tablespoons buttermilk

- 1 ½ tablespoons poppy seeds

- 1 tablespoon vanilla extract

- 1 ½ teaspoons baking powder

Preparation

1. Make the candied kumquats: Prepare an ice bath in a medium bowl and set to the side with a medium fine-mesh strainer.

2. Bring a small pot of water to a boil, then add the kumquats and blanch for 1 minute. Immediately pour through the fine-mesh strainer, then set the strainer with the kumquats in the ice bath to shock (this will help keep the bright orange color of the kumquats).

3. In the same small pot, combine the sugar and water and cook over medium heat until the sugar dissolves, 2–3 minutes. Add the kumquats and reduce the heat to low. Simmer for 20–30 minutes, until the kumquats are soft and translucent. Use a small strainer or fork to remove the kumquats from the syrup and transfer to a wire rack to dry, making

sure that none of the slices are touching. Let cool completely. Set the pot aside.

4. Make the citrus poppy muffins: Preheat the oven to 375°F (190°C). Generously grease a standard or mini muffin tin with nonstick spray.

5. Zest the kumquats, tangerines, and Meyer lemons into a small bowl. Set the citrus aside.

6. In the bowl of a stand mixer fitted with the paddle attachment, cream together the butter, 1 cup sugar, the salt, and citrus zest on medium-high speed until light and fluffy, about 2 minutes. Scrape down the sides of the bowl.

7. Reduce the mixer speed to low speed and add the eggs and egg yolks, 1 at a time, mixing to incorporate between each addition.

8. Turn the mixer off and add the flour, buttermilk, poppy seeds, vanilla, and baking powder. Mix on

low speed until just barely combined; do not overmix.

9. Use an ice cream scoop to scoop batter into the prepared muffin tin, filling each cavity half to three quarters of the way full.

10. Bake the muffins until the edges are golden brown and a toothpick inserted into the center comes out clean, 12–15 minutes for regular muffins or 8–11 minutes for mini muffins.

11. Meanwhile, add the remaining 5 tablespoons of sugar, the zested kumquats and tangerines, and juice of the zested Meyer lemons to a blender. Blend on low speed until the mixture is a chunky purée.

12. Pour the purée into the same pot used to candy the kumquats. Bring to a simmer over low heat and cook for about 5 minutes, until the sugar is

dissolved. Remove from the heat and let steep until ready to use.

13. Once the muffins are done, remove from the oven. Set a wire rack over a baking sheet and place this upside down on top of the muffins. Carefully flip the upside down to turn the muffins out of the pan while still hot, then quickly flip them right-side-up on the rack. Strain the citrus purée to remove the solids, then use a pastry brush to brush a thick layer of the purée on top of each muffin while they are still warm. Before the glaze dries, decorate the tops of the muffins with the candied kumquats.

14. The muffins are best the day they are made, but any leftovers will keep tightly wrapped at room temperature for up to 2 days.

15. Enjoy!

Triple Chocolate Trifle

Ingredients

for 2 servings

Chocolate Pudding

• 1 cup whole milk (240 mL)

• 1 can cream

• ½ cup granulated sugar (100 g)

• ¼ cup cocoa powder (25 g)

• 3 tablespoons cornstarch

• ¼ teaspoon kosher salt

• 1 tablespoon unsalted butter, room temperature

• 1 teaspoon vanilla extract

Chocolate Whipped Cream

• 1 cup heavy whipping cream (240 mL)

• ¼ cup powdered sugar (25 g)

• 2 tablespoons unsweetened cocoa powder

Dark Chocolate Ganache

• ¼ cup heavy cream (60 mL)

• 3 tablespoons dark chocolate chip

Assembly

• 7 oz chocolate pound cake (200 g), cut into 1/2 in

• ½ cup chocolate sandwich cookie (60 g), finely crushed

• ½ cup chocolate caramel candy (100 g), chopped

• fresh raspberry, for garnish

• fresh mint leaf, for garnish

• chocolate spoon, optional, for serving

Preparation

1. Make the pudding: In a medium pot, combine the milk, table cream, sugar, cocoa powder, cornstarch, and salt and whisk together until evenly incorporated. Cook over medium-high heat, whisking constantly, until starting to thicken and bubble up, about 5 minutes.

2. Remove the pot from the heat and whisk in the butter and vanilla. Strain the pudding through a fine-mesh sieve into a medium bowl. Cover with plastic wrap, pressing directly against the surface of the pudding to prevent a skin from forming. Chill in the refrigerator for at least 2 hours, or overnight.

3. Make the whipped cream: In a medium bowl, combine the heavy cream, powdered sugar, and cocoa powder. Whip with an electric hand mixer on high speed until stiff peaks form, 3–4 minutes, scraping down the sides of the bowl as needed. Transfer the whipped cream to a piping bag fitted with a large tip and chill in the refrigerator until ready to use.

4. Make the chocolate ganache: Add heavy cream to a microwave-safe liquid measuring cup. Microwave for 1 minute, until very hot. Add the chocolate chips and let sit for 2 minutes, then stir until smooth. Transfer to a piping bag fitted with a small tip. Set aside until ready to use.

5. Assemble the trifles: Transfer the chocolate pudding to a piping bag fitted with a large tip.

6. Add about ½ cup of the pound cake cubes to the bottom of each jar, pressing down to compact. Pipe

about ¼ cup of chocolate pudding and ¼ cup of the whipped cream on top. Sprinkle 2–3 tablespoons of crushed chocolate sandwich cookies and 2 tablespoons chocolate caramel candy bars on top. Repeat to make a second layer with the remaining ingredients. Finish with a drizzle of chocolate ganache and garnish with fresh raspberries and a sprig of mint. Serve with chocolate spoons.

7. Enjoy!

Marshmallow Sweet Potato Pie

Ingredients

for 6 servings

• 3 large egg whites, room temperature

- 1 cup marshmallow fluff (85 g)

- 1 store-bought sweet potato pie

Preparation

1. Preheat the oven to 350°F (180°C).

2. Beat the egg whites in a large bowl with an electric hand mixer on high speed until soft peaks form, 2–3 minutes.

3. Gradually add the marshmallow fluff and continue beating until stiff, glossy peaks form, 2–3 minutes.

4. Dollop the topping on top of the sweet potato pie and swirl into peaks.

5. Bake the pie until the meringue has browned, 10–12 minutes.

6. Let cool before serving.

7. Enjoy!

Zucchini Almond Bread

Ingredients

for 6 slices

Bread

• 8 oz crushed pineapple (225 g), 1 can, with juice

• 3 eggs

• 1 cup vegetable oil (240 mL), or oil of your choice

• 1 cup sugar (200 g)

• 1 cup brown sugar (220 g)

• 2 cups zucchini (300 g), grated

• 3 teaspoons vanilla

• 3 cups flour (375 g)

• 1 teaspoon salt

• 1 teaspoon baking soda

• 3 teaspoons cinnamon

• ½ teaspoon nutmeg

• 1 cup chopped almond (100 g)

• thinly sliced almond, for topping

Glaze

• ¼ tablespoon vanilla

• ½ cup powdered sugar (80 g)

• 1 tablespoon milk

Preparation

1. Mix all of the dry **Ingredients** (flour, salt, baking soda, cinnamon, nutmeg, chopped almonds) in a bowl, and set aside.

2. Preheated oven at 350ºF (175ºC).

3. In a new bowl, combine pineapple, eggs, vegetable oil, sugar, brown sugar, zucchini, and vanilla, and mix well.

4. Pour the dry **Ingredients** gradually into the wet **Ingredients** bowl, and mix them until smooth.

5. Spray your baking pan and pour in the mixture, top with sliced almonds.

6. Bake for 60 minutes (times may vary depending on oven), and check for doneness with a toothpick.

7. While baking, mix your glaze **Ingredients** together until smooth.

8. Let the bread cool down, drizzle with the glaze!

9. Enjoy!

Tri-Color Fruit Mousse

Ingredients

for 4 servings

Blackberry Layer

• 1 tablespoon cold water

• 1 teaspoon unflavored gelatin powder

• ½ cup frozen blackberry pulp (75 g), thawed

- 1 tablespoon blackberry powder, optional

- ¾ cup heavy cream (180 mL)

- ½ cup sweetened condensed milk (120 mL)

Guava Layer

- 1 tablespoon cold water

- 1 teaspoon unflavored gelatin powder

- ½ cup frozen guava pulp (130 g), thawed

- 1 tablespoon guava powder, optional

- ¾ cup heavy cream (180 mL)

- ½ cup sweetened condensed milk (120 mL)

Passion Fruit Layer

- 1 tablespoon cold water

- 1 teaspoon unflavored gelatin powder

- ½ cup frozen passion fuit pulp (130 g), thawed

- 1 tablespoon passion fruit powder, optional

- ¾ cup heavy cream (180 mL)

- ½ cup sweetened condensed milk (120 mL)

For Topping

- 4 tablespoons passion fruit pulp

- 6 blackberries, halved lengthwise

Preparation

1. Make the blackberry layer: In a medium bowl, whisk together the water and gelatin.

2. In a small saucepan over medium-high heat, bring the blackberry pulp to a boil. Remove the pot from the heat and pour the pulp over the gelatin.

Whisk to melt the gelatin completely. Add the blackberry powder, if using, and whisk until fully incorporated. Set aside to cool while you whip the cream.

3. In a large bowl, combine the heavy cream and sweetened condensed milk. Using an electric hand mixer on medium-high speed, whip until medium peaks form. Pour in the blackberry pulp mixture and fold with a rubber spatula completely combined.

4. Divide the mixture evenly between 4 10-ounce glasses. Refrigerate while you make the guava layer.

5. Make the guava layer: In a medium bowl, whisk together the water and gelatin.

6. In a small saucepan over medium-high heat, bring the guava pulp to a boil. Remove the pot from the heat and pour the pulp over the gelatin. Whisk

to melt the gelatin completely. Add the guava powder, if using, and whisk until fully incorporated. Set aside to cool while you whip the cream.

7. In a large bowl, combine the heavy cream and sweetened condensed milk. Using an electric hand mixer on medium-high speed, whip until medium peaks form. Pour in the guava pulp mixture and fold with a rubber spatula completely combined

8. Divide the mixture evenly between the glasses, layering on top of the blackberry layer. Refrigerate while you make the passion fruit layer.

9. Make the passion fruit layer: In a medium bowl, whisk together the water and gelatin.

10. In a small saucepan over medium-high heat, bring the passion fruit pulp to a boil. Remove the pot from the heat and pour the pulp over the gelatin. Whisk to melt the gelatin completely. Add

the passion fruit powder, if using, and whisk until fully incorporated. Set aside to cool while you whip the cream.

11. In a large bowl, combine the heavy cream and sweetened condensed milk. Using an electric hand mixer on medium-high speed, whip until medium peaks form. Pour in the passion fruit pulp mixture and fold with a rubber spatula completely combined.

12. Divide the mixture evenly between the glasses, layering on top of the guava layer. Refrigerate for at least 15 minutes, and up to 3 days, until the mousse sets completely.

13. Top each mousse with 1 tablespoon of passion fruit pulp and 3 blackberry halves.

14. Enjoy!

Frozen Waffle

Ingredients

for 12 servings

• 2 cups all purpose flour (250 g)

• ⅓ cup Dutch-process cocoa powder (35 g), sifted, plus 2 tablespoons

• ½ cup granulated sugar (55 g), divided, plus 2 tablespoons

• 2 teaspoons baking powder

• 1 teaspoon baking soda

• 1 teaspoon espresso powder

• ½ teaspoon kosher salt

• 2 cups Planet Oat Oatmilk (480 mL)

• 1 tablespoon white vinegar

• ¼ cup vegetable oil (60 mL)

• 2 large eggs, separated

• nonstick cooking spray, for greasing

• 3 pt Planet Oat® Vanilla Non-Dairy Dessert (1.3 g)

• melted chocolate, for drizzling or dipping

• rainbow sprinkle, for topping

• peanut, chopped, for topping

Preparation

1. Preheat the waffle iron according to the manufacturer's instructions.

2. In a large bowl, whisk together the flour, cocoa powder, ½ cup sugar, the baking powder, baking soda, espresso powder, and salt.

3. In a medium bowl, whisk together the Planet Oat Oatmilk and the vinegar. Let sit for 5 minutes, then mix in vegetable oil and egg yolks.

4. Add the wet **Ingredients** to the dry ingredients, stirring until just combined. Do not overmix; a few lumps are okay.

5. In a medium bowl, whisk the egg whites with the remaining 2 tablespoons of sugar until frothy and doubled in volume, about 5 minutes.

6. Fold the egg whites into the waffle batter until just combined.

7. Grease the waffle iron with nonstick spray. Cook the waffles according to the waffle iron instructions. Transfer the waffles to a wire rack, arranging in a single layer, and let cool to room temperature.

8. Line a baking sheet with parchment paper. Transfer the waffles to the prepared baking sheet and freeze for 15–30 minutes, until cold.

9. Remove the Planet Oat® Vanilla Non-Dairy Dessert from the freezer and let sit for 10–15 minutes, until softened.

10. Top a waffle with 4 scoops of Planet Oat® Vanilla Non-Dairy Dessert in each quadrant, then place a second waffle on top to form a sandwich. Repeat with the remaining ingredients.

11. Return the waffle sandwiches to the baking sheet and freeze for 3–4 hours, until frozen solid.

12. Remove from the freezer and cut each waffle sandwich into quarters to make 4 smaller sandwiches. Dip in or drizzle with melted chocolate, or roll the edges in sprinkles or chopped peanuts. Freeze until ready to serve.

13. Enjoy!

Gingerbread Cinnamon Rolls

Ingredients

for 8 rolls

Dough

- 2 cups all purpose flour (250 g)

- 1 ½ cups whole wheat flour (185 g)

- ½ cup granulated sugar (100 g)

- 2 teaspoons instant yeast

- 2 teaspoons kosher salt

- 1 ½ teaspoons ground ginger

- 4 large eggs

- 2 sticks unsalted butter, melted

- ⅓ cup whole milk (80 g)

- 1 tablespoon molasses

Filling

- 1 stick unsalted butter, softened

- ½ cup light brown sugar (100 g)

- 1 tablespoon molasses

- 2 teaspoons McCormick® ground ginger

- 1 teaspoon McCormick® Ground Cinnamon

- ½ teaspoon freshly grated nutmeg

- ½ teaspoon McCormick® Ground Cloves

- ½ teaspoon McCormick® five-spice powder

- ¼ teaspoon kosher salt

Icing

- 4 oz cream cheese (110 g)

- ½ stick unsalted butter, softened

- ¼ teaspoon kosher salt

- 1 ½ cups powdered sugar (165 g)

- ½ cup gingersnaps (50 g), crushed

Preparation

1. Make the dough: In a large bowl, whisk together the all-purpose and whole wheat flours, sugar, yeast, salt, and ground ginger.

2. In the bowl of a stand mixer fitted with the dough hook, combine the eggs, butter, milk, and molasses.

Mix on medium-low speed to combine. Add the flour mixture and mix on medium speed until a shaggy mass forms. Reduce the speed to medium-low and continue mixing until the dough begins to climb the hook, about 15 minutes. The dough will be very wet, but it will come together as it rests. Cover the bowl with plastic wrap or a kitchen towel and let rest in a warm place until doubled in size, about 2 hours.

3. Lightly wet your hands and gently punch down the dough (wetting your hands will help prevent the dough from sticking when you punch it down). Cover the bowl again and transfer to the refrigerator so the dough can stiffen, at least 1 hour, or up to overnight.

4. Make the filling: In a medium bowl, combine the butter, brown sugar, molasses, ginger, cinnamon,

nutmeg, cloves, five-spice, and salt. Use a fork to mash together until smooth.

5. Turn the dough out onto a lightly floured surface and roll out to ¼-inch-thick rectangle. Spread the filling across the dough, all the way to the edges. Starting from a long end, roll the dough into a log. Trim the ends, then slice the log crosswise into 8 pieces.

6. Place the rolls in a 9-inch round springform pan. Cover with a kitchen towel and let proof in a warm place until doubled in size, about 2 hours.

7. Preheat the oven to 350°F (180°C).

8. Uncover the buns and bake until golden brown and cooked through, about 30 minutes. Remove from the oven and let cool slightly.

9. Make the icing: In a large bowl with an electric hand mixer (or in the bowl of a stand mixer fitted

with the whisk attachment), cream together the cream cheese, butter, and salt on medium speed until smooth, about 1 minute. Add the powdered sugar and continue mixing until creamy, about 1 minute.

10. Spread the icing over the cinnamon rolls and sprinkle the crushed gingersnap cookies on top.

11. Enjoy!

THYROID RESET RECIPES FOR LUNCH

Black Bean Soup

Ingredients

for 6 servings

• 2 tablespoons olive oil

• 2 cups diced yellow onion

• 1 cup chopped celery

• 1 cup chopped carrot

• 1 red bell pepper, seeded and diced

• 1 teaspoon kosher salt

• 1 teaspoon freshly ground black pepper

• 4 cloves garlic, minced

• 1 jalapeño, seeded and diced

• 2 tablespoons ground cumin

• 60 oz black beans (1.75 kg), drained and rinsed

• 4 cups vegetable stock (960 mL)

• 1 dried bay leaf

For Serving

• diced avocado

• crumbled queso fresco

• chopped fresh cilantro

Preparation

1. Heat the olive oil in a large stockpot or Dutch oven over medium-high heat until the oil begins to shimmer. Add the onion, celery, carrot, and bell pepper. Cook for 4-5 minutes, stirring occasionally, until the vegetables begin to soften.

2. Add salt, pepper, garlic, and jalapeño and continue to cook for an additional 10 minutes, until the vegetables are tender and the onion is translucent.

3. Add the cumin, black beans, vegetable stock, and bay leaf. Bring to a boil, then reduce the heat to low. Cover the pot and simmer for 30 minutes, until the beans are very tender.

4. Remove the bay leaf. Transfer about 4 cups (900 g) of the soup to a blender and carefully purée until smooth, leaving the top vent of the blender open and covering with a kitchen towel to prevent the soup from splattering.

5. Pour the blended soup back into the pot and stir to incorporate. Keep warm over low heat until ready to serve.

6. Ladle the soup into bowls and garnish with avocado, queso fresco, and cilantro.

7. Enjoy!

Butternut Squash Soup

Ingredients

for 6 servings

• 2 lb medium butternut squash (910 g), peeled, seeded, roughly chopped

• 1 medium yellow onion, roughly chopped

- 4 cloves garlic

- olive oil, to taste

- 3 cups vegetable broth (720 mL)

- ½ teaspoon ground ginger

- ½ teaspoon ground cumin

- ½ teaspoon ground coriander

- ½ teaspoon paprika

- ⅛ teaspoon cayenne pepper

- 1 ½ teaspoons sea salt

- ¼ teaspoon black pepper

- ½ teaspoon fresh thyme

- ¼ cup coconut milk (60 mL)

Optional Garnishes

• pumpkin seed

• fresh chive, chopped

Preparation

1. Add the butternut squash, onion, and garlic to a slow cooker. Drizzle with olive oil and add vegetable broth, ginger, cumin, coriander, paprika, cayenne, salt, and pepper.

2. Cover and cook on high heat for 4 hours.

3. Using a hand blender, blend the **Ingredients** until smooth, or transfer to a standard blender or food processor and carefully puree.

4. Add the thyme and coconut milk and blend to incorporate.

5. Garnish with pumpkin seeds and chives, if desired.

6. Enjoy!

Roasted Butternut Squash Soup

Ingredients

for 8 servings

• 2 butternut squashes, peeled, seeded and cut into 2 in (5 cm) cubes

• 4 tablespoons olive oil, divided

• 2 ½ teaspoons kosher salt, divided

• 4 tablespoons unsalted butter, divided

• 1 large white onion, diced

- 4 cloves garlic, minced

- 1 tablespoon fresh sage, chopped

- 1 cup dry white wine (240 mL)

- 8 cups vegetable broth (1.9 L)

- ½ cup heavy cream (120 mL), plus more for serving

- ½ cup walnuts (50 g), toasted

- 8 teaspoons chive oil, for serving

Chive Oil

- 2 cups ice (280 g)

- 8 cups water (1.9 L), divided

- ½ oz fresh chives (15 g)

- ¾ cup neutral oil (180 mL)

Preparation

1. Preheat the oven to 400°F (200°C).

2. In a large bowl, toss the butternut squash with 2 tablespoons of olive oil and 1 teaspoon of salt until well coated. Spread the squash in a single layer on an unlined baking sheet.

3. Roast the squash for 60–70 minutes, until completely tender and just beginning to brown on the edges.

4. Once the squash has been roasting for 40 minutes, start the soup: In a large stock pot, melt 2 tablespoons of butter and the remaining 2 tablespoons of olive oil over medium heat. Add the onion and season with 1 teaspoon of salt. Sauté for 8–10 minutes, until the onion is translucent and fragrant.

5. Add the garlic and sage and stir to combine. Sauté for another 8–10 minutes, until the onions are beginning to caramelize slightly. Add the white wine and cook for 2–4 minutes, until reduced by about half.

6. Add the squash to the pot, along with the vegetable broth. Increase the heat to medium-high and bring to a boil. Cover the pot and reduce the heat to medium-low. Simmer for 15–20 minutes, until the squash is completely broken down.

7. Remove the pot from the heat. Stir in the heavy cream and remaining 2 tablespoons of butter. Using an immersion blender, blend until the soup is completely smooth and creamy. Season with the remaining ½ teaspoon of salt, plus more to taste.

8. Ladle the hot soup into bowls. Top with the toasted walnuts, a drizzle of heavy cream, and a drizzle of chive oil.

9. To make the chive oil, combine the ice and 3 cups (720 ml) of water in a medium bowl. Set near the stovetop.

10. Add the remaining 3 cups (720 ml) of water to a small saucepan and bring to a simmer over medium-high heat. Add the chives to the simmering water and blanch for 30 seconds, then strain. Transfer the strainer directly to the ice bath to halt the cooking process. Let the chives cool for 1 minute, then drain on paper towels.

11. Add the chives and oil to a liquid measuring cup or other tall, narrow container. Using an immersion blender, blend until the chives are completely broken down. Do not overblend, as the chives can turn brown.

12. Place a damp paper towel inside a strainer and set over a medium bowl. Pour the chive oil through the strainer to remove any remaining solids.

13. Use the chive oil as desired. It will keep in an airtight container in the refrigerator for up to 3 months.

14. Enjoy!

Mexican Red Pork Tamales

Ingredients

for 16 servings

For Wrapping

• 1 bag dry corn husks

• hot water, for soaking

Tamales

• 2 roma tomatoes

- ½ small white onion

- 2 dried guajillo chiles

- 2 dried pasilla chiles

- 2 cloves garlic

- 4 cups water (960 mL), divided, plus 1 tablespoon

- 2 teaspoons salt, plus more to taste

- pepper, to taste

- ½ tablespoon ground cumin

- 2 tablespoons canola oil

- 3 lb pork shoulder (1.5 kg), cubed

- 1 teaspoon baking soda

- 1 teaspoon baking powder

- ¾ cup lard (145 g)

- 2 lb fresh corn masa (905 g)

- salsa verde, for serving

Preparation

1. Place the dry corn husks in a baking dish. Pour hot water over the husks to cover. Weigh the husks down so they are completely submerged and let soak for 2 hours, or until pliable.

2. Add the tomatoes, onion, guajillos, pasillas, garlic, and 4 cups (960 ml) of water to a small pot. Cover, bring to a boil, and cook for 10 minutes, or until the vegetables have softened.

3. Transfer the vegetables to a blender, Add salt and pepper to taste, the cumin, and about ½ cup (60 ml) of the cooking liquid. Blend until smooth. Set aside.

4. Heat the canola oil in a large skillet over medium-high heat. Add the pork and season with salt and pepper. Fry the pork until well-browned and most of the fat has evaporated. Drain any excess fat, if necessary.

5. Add the sauce to the pan with the pork, bring to a boil, cover, and let simmer until tender, about 1 hour. Remove from the heat and let cool.

6. In a small bowl, combine the baking soda, baking powder, and 1 tablespoon water. Stir to dissolve, then set aside.

7. Add the lard to a large bowl. With an electric hand mixer, whip the lard until light and fluffy, about 5 minutes.

8. Add the masa and baking soda mixture and mix with your hands until smooth, about 5 minutes. It should be spreadable but still hold its shape.

9. Drain the soaked corn husks.

10. Place 1 husk on a clean surface and add 1-2 tablespoons of masa to the center of the husk. Spread with the back of the spoon to about ¼ inch (¾ cm) from the edges.

11. Place 1 tablespoon of meat in the center. Roll the corn husk over the filling from left to right and fold the top down to create a little pocket. Set aside. Repeat with the remaining ingredients.

12. Place the tamales, open ends up, in a steamer basket set over a large pot of boiling water. Cover with a clean kitchen towel and the lid. Let steam for 1 hour, then turn off the heat and let the tamales rest for 1 hour more.

13. Unwrap the tamales and serve with salsa verde.

14. Enjoy!

Cheddar-Crusted & Bacon Broccoli Quiche

Ingredients

for 8 servings

• 2 ½ cups shredded cheddar cheese (250 g), divided

• 1 cup unsalted butter (230 g), 2 sticks, room temperature

• 2 cups all-purpose flour (250 g), plus more for dusting

• 1 tablespoon paprika

• 1 tablespoon garlic powder

• 2 ½ teaspoons salt, divided

• 5 tablespoons ice water

- 4 strips bacon

- 2 cups small broccoli floret (300 g)

- 6 large eggs

- 1 cup milk (240 mL)

- ½ teaspoon pepper

Preparation

1. Preheat the oven to 350°F (180°C).

2. Add 2 cups (200 g) of cheddar cheese and the butter to a large bowl. Mix to combine with an electric hand mixer or stand mixer.

3. Add the flour, paprika, garlic powder, and 2 teaspoons salt and mix well. Add 3 tablespoons of ice water and mix. Add the remaining ice water 1 tablespoon at a time. The dough should hold together when pinched, but crumble apart if you

break it up in your hand. If it seems too dry, add a bit more ice water.

4. Transfer the dough to a clean surface and knead with your hands until it comes together. Shape the dough into a disc, then wrap in plastic wrap and chill in the refrigerator for 30 minutes.

5. Lightly flour a clean surface and roll out the dough into a circle about ⅛ inch (8 mm) thick. Carefully transfer the crust to a 9½-inch (24-cm) glass pie dish.

6. Trim the edges (save the trimmings to make crackers!). Poke holes in the bottom of the crust with a fork, then use the tines to crimp the edges. Line the dough with parchment paper and fill with pie weights.

7. Bake for 30 minutes, until the edges are crisp.

8. While the crust is baking, prepare the fillings. In a large skillet over medium-high heat, cook the bacon until crisp, 5-7 minutes. Using tongs, remove the bacon from the skillet and let drain on paper towels until cool enough to handle.

9. Add the broccoli to the skillet and cook until lightly browned, about 5 minutes. Remove the pan from the heat.

10. Chop the bacon.

11. Remove the pie weights from the crust, then add the broccoli and chopped bacon to the center. Sprinkle with the remaining shredded cheddar cheese.

12. In a medium bowl, lightly beat the eggs. Add the milk, remaining ½ teaspoon salt, and the pepper. Whisk to combine.

13. Pour the egg mixture over the fillings in the crust.

14. Bake for 35-40 minutes, or until the eggs are set and the top is lightly browned. Cover the edges with tinfoil if they are starting to burn.

15. Let the quiche cool for 15 minutes before slicing and serving.

16. Enjoy!

Pear Butter Chicken And Waffles

Ingredients

for 4 servings

Pear Butter

- 3 barlett pears, peeled, cored, and cut into ½-inch(1.2 cm) cubes

- ½ cup water (120 mL)

- ½ tablespoon cinnamon

- ½ teaspoon ground nutmeg

- ¼ teaspoon ground allspice

- ¼ teaspoon ground cloves

- ¾ cup sugar (150 g)

Waffles

- 2 cups all purpose flour (250 g)

- ½ cup sugar (100 g)

- ¼ teaspoon kosher salt

- 4 teaspoons baking powder

- ½ cup vegetable oil (120 mL)

- ¾ cup heavy cream (180 mL)

- 1 cup milk (240 mL)

- 1 tablespoon vanilla extract

- 2 large eggs, beaten

- nonstick cooking spray, for greasing

Whipped Cream

- 1 cup heavy cream (240 mL)

- 1 teaspoon cinnamon

- 1 ½ tablespoons powdered sugar

- fresh mint sprig, for garnish

Chicken

• 6 cups neutral oil (1.4 L), such as vegetable oil, for frying

• 4 boneless skinless chicken breasts, cut into 2-inch (5 cm) wide strips

• 1 ½ teaspoons lemon pepper

• 1 ½ teaspoons kosher salt

• 1 teaspoon Ac'cent® seasoning

• 1 ½ cups all purpose flour (185 g)

Preparation

1. Make the pear butter: Add the pears, water, cinnamon, nutmeg, allspice, cloves, and sugar to a medium saucepan and stir to coat the pears. Bring to a simmer over medium-high heat, then reduce the heat to medium-low and cook, stirring occasionally, until the pears are tender, 35–40

minutes. Remove the pot from the heat. Using a potato masher, mash the pears until broken down to the consistency of a chunky applesauce. Set aside.

2. Make the waffles: Preheat a waffle iron according to the manufacturer's instructions.

3. In a large bowl, whisk together the flour, sugar, salt, baking powder, oil, cream, milk, and vanilla until smooth. Mix in the beaten eggs.

4. Ladle a scant ½ cup (55 G) of the waffle batter per waffle into the preheated waffle iron. Cook for 3–4 minutes, or until golden brown and cooked through. Repeat with the remaining batter. Keep the waffles warm in a low-heated oven until ready to use.

5. Make the whipped cream: Add the heavy cream, cinnamon, and powdered sugar to a large bowl.

Whip with an electric hand mixer on medium speed until stiff peaks form, about 2 minutes. Refrigerate until ready to use.

6. Make the chicken: Heat the vegetable oil in a large, high-walled skillet over medium-high heat until it reaches 350°F (180°C).

7. In a large bowl, season the chicken with the lemon pepper, salt, and Ac'cent seasoning, tossing to coat well. Add the flour to a medium bowl. Dredge the chicken in the flour, shaking off any excess.

8. Working in batches, gently lower the chicken into the hot oil and fry until golden brown, 6–8 minutes, or until the internal temperature reaches 165°F (75°C). Remove from the oil using tongs or a slotted spoon and transfer to a paper-towel lined plate to drain while you fry the remaining chicken.

9. Cut the waffles into triangles and arrange 3 on each plate. Top with 2 tablespoons of pear butter, 3 fried chicken strips, and a dollop of whipped cream. Garnish with a sprig of mint.

10. Enjoy!

Vegetable Rose Herb Cheese Tart

Ingredients

for 12 servings

Crust

• 60 butter crackers

• ½ teaspoon kosher salt

• 1 teaspoon black pepper

• ⅓ cup parmesan cheese (35 g), grated

• 2 tablespoons melted butter

• 1 large egg, beaten

Filling

• 1 ½ packages cream cheese, softened (8 ounce packages . 225 gram)

• ⅓ cup sour cream (80 g)

• 1 large egg

• ¼ cup grated parmesan cheese (25 g)

• ½ teaspoon kosher salt

• ½ teaspoon black pepper

• ¾ teaspoon garlic powder

• ¼ cup fresh chives (10 g), chopped

- ¼ cup fresh dill (10 g), chopped

- 1 tablespoon fresh thyme leaf, finely chopped

Vegetable Roses

- 2 medium zucchinis, ends trimmed

- 8 rainbow carrots, peeled and ends trimmed

- 2 tablespoons olive oil

- ½ teaspoon kosher salt

- ½ teaspoon black pepper

Preparation

1. Preheat oven to 350°F (180°C).

2. Add the crackers to the bowl of a food processor. Pulse until finely ground. Add the melted butter, salt, pepper, Parmesan cheese, melted butter and

egg. Pulse until combined, scraping the sides to make sure everything is incorporated.

3. Transfer the crust mixture to a 9-inch (22 cm) tart pan and place on a baking sheet. Use a spatula and your hands to press the crust into the bottoms and sides of the pan in an even layer.

4. Bake the crust for 12–14 minutes, until the edges just begin to brown. Let cool completely.

5. Make the filling: In a large bowl, use an electric hand mixer to beat the cream cheese until light and fluffy. Add the sour cream and beat to combine. Add the egg and beat until incorporated. Use a spatula to fold in the grated Parmesan cheese, salt, pepper, garlic powder, chives, dill, and thyme.

6. Carefully pour the filling into the tart crust. Use an offset spatula to smooth the top in an even layer.

7. Make the vegetable roses: Using a vegetable peeler, shave the zucchini and carrots into wide ribbons. Place in a large bowl and microwave for 1 minute to release excess water and make the ribbons more pliable.

8. Rolling the vegetable ribbons tightly into roses, using 1–4 ribbons per rose for varying sizes.

9. Starting in the center, nestle the vegetable roses into the filling, working to about ½ inch (1 ¼ cm) from the edge of the tart. Brush the tops of the roses with the olive oil and sprinkle with salt and pepper.

10. Transfer the tart to the oven and bake for about 40 minutes, until the edges of the filling are golden and the center looks set.

11. Let the tart cool completely. Slice and serve, or refrigerate and bring back to room temperature for at least 1 hour before serving.

12. Enjoy!

King Cake

Ingredients

for 12 servings

Dough

• 1 stick unsalted butter, melted

• ¾ cup milk (180 mL), lukewarm

• 2 large eggs, room temperature

• 3 ½ cups all purpose flour (435 g), plus more for dusting

• ¼ cup granulated sugar (50 g)

- 2 ¼ teaspoons instant yeast

- 1 teaspoon kosher salt

- 1 teaspoon lemon zest

- ¼ teaspoon freshly grated nutmeg

- nonstick cooking spray, for greasing

Filling

- ¾ stick unsalted butter

- ¾ cup brown sugar (150 g)

- 2 teaspoons ground cinnamon

- ¼ teaspoon kosher salt

Egg Wash

- 1 large egg

• 1 tablespoon milk

Glaze

• 2 ½ cups powdered sugar (275 g)

• 2 tablespoons milk

• 1 tablespoon lemon juice

• 1 teaspoon vanilla extract

Topping

• green sparkling sugar

• yellow sparkling sugar

• purple sparkling sugar

Special Equipment

• 1 large dried bean

Preparation

1. Make the dough: In the bowl of a stand mixer fitted with the dough hook, combine the melted butter, milk, eggs, flour, granulated sugar, yeast, salt, lemon zest, and nutmeg. Mix on medium-low speed for 7–8 minutes, scraping down the sides of the bowl as needed, until the dough is silky smooth.

2. Shape the dough into a ball. Grease a medium bowl with nonstick spray, transfer the dough to the bowl, and turn to coat. Cover with plastic wrap and let rise in a warm place for 1 hour, until about 1½ times its original size.

3. While the dough is rising, make the filling: In a separate medium bowl, combine the softened butter, brown sugar, cinnamon, and salt. Mix with a fork until thoroughly combined.

4. Make the egg wash: In a small bowl, beat together the egg and milk with a fork until thoroughly combined.

5. Assemble the king cake: Line a baking sheet with parchment paper.

6. Turn the dough out onto a lightly floured surface. Lightly flour the top and roll out to a 10 x 22-inch rectangle. Use a pizza cutter or sharp knife to cut the rectangle lengthwise into 3 even strips.

7. Use a small offset or silicone spatula to spread the filling evenly over half of the long side of each strip, leaving the other half of each strip uncovered. Brush the uncovered dough lightly with the egg wash. Starting from the side with the filling, roll each strip into a log and position seam-side down. Press one end of each of the logs together, then braid the logs into a single long strand. Bring the ends of the braid together to make a ring, pressing

together to secure. Carefully transfer the ring to the prepared baking sheet, making sure to maintain the large opening in the center. Cover with plastic wrap and let proof in a warm place for 30-45 minutes, until the dough is pillowy to the touch.

8. Preheat the oven to 375°F (190°C).

9. Brush the ring with egg wash. Bake for 30–32 minutes, until golden brown. Remove from the oven and let cool completely, about 1 hour.

10. Decorate the cake: Carefully flip the cake upside down and use a sharp knife to create a small slit in the bottom. Hide the plastic baby in the slit. Flip the cake right-side up.

11. Make the glaze: In a medium bowl, whisk together the powdered sugar, 2 tablespoons milk, the lemon juice, and vanilla until smooth. Add the

remaining milk as needed to create a thick, yet pourable glaze.

12. Pour the glaze evenly over the top of the cake. While the glaze is still wet, decorate with alternating stripes of green, yellow, and purple sparkling sugar. Let the icing set for at least 30 minutes before slicing and serving.

13. Enjoy!

Frankenstein's Arm Charcuterie

Ingredients

for 8 servings

• 10 oz goat cheese (290 g), room temperature

• 8 oz cream cheese (225 g), room temperature

- ½ bunch fresh flat-leaf parsley

- ½ cup fresh chives (20 g), thinly sliced

- ½ teaspoon freshly ground black pepper

- 4 string cheeses

- 8 slices prosciutto

- 3 tablespoons pesto, chilled

- 2 large green olives, pitted

For Serving

- Crudité

- cracker

Preparation

1. In a large bowl, combine the goat cheese, cream cheese, parsley, chives, and pepper. Mix with an

electric hand mixer or a spatula until the herbs are evenly distributed. Cover and refrigerate until ready to use.

2. Tape a piece of parchment paper to a cutting board and trace your hand and 3 inches down your wrist. Lay a sheet of plastic wrap over the parchment.

3. Cut 1 string cheese in half crosswise; these pieces will be the thumb and pinky. Trim 2 of the string cheeses to be about 2 inches long; these will be the index and ring fingers. Keep the remaining string cheese whole. Wrap each piece of string cheese in prosciutto, making sure to cover the ends that will be the fingertips.

4. Using a 1-ounce scoop, scoop 6 portions of the goat cheese mixture onto the wrist area of the traced arm. Add another 4 scoops to the back of the hand area. Use an offset spatula to smooth out the

scoops to make a smooth surface. Use the tip of the spatula or the back of a spoon to create a ½-inch-deep divot down the center of the wrist and a well in the center of the hand. Spread some of the goat cheese mixture down each finger tracing. This will help secure the string cheese fingers and create a smoother look. Fill the divot and well with the pesto, being careful not to spill over the sides. If the cheese is becoming too warm at this point, lightly cover with plastic wrap and refrigerate for 30 minutes before proceeding.

5. Place each prosciutto-wrapped string cheese on their respective finger tracing, pressing down onto the goat cheese to secure.

6. Add 3 scoops of the goat cheese mixture to the wrist area in a single line and 3 more scoops to the back of the hand area. Smooth with the offset spatula to create the wrist and arm, covering the

pesto. Make sure to spread the goat cheese mixture over where the string cheeses attach to the hand to create a smooth look, using your fingers as needed. You may have some excess cheese mixture leftover, depending on the size of your tracing. Fill in any patches with more of the goat cheese mixture and shape the cheese to create a realistic hand shape.

7. Cover the entire hand and wrist with the remaining prosciutto. You may want to tear the prosciutto into smaller pieces for a more realistic effect.

8. Cut the olives into quarters. Square off one end of each quarter and leave the other end pointy to resemble a fingernail. Trim each "fingernail" to fit the respective finger you will be placing it on (for example, make the thumbnail slightly larger than the index fingernail, and so on). You will only need 5 pieces total.

9. Cut ½-inch divots into each fingertip. Add a tiny bit of the remaining goat cheese mixture to each divot, then press the olive fingernails into their respective fingers.

10. Cover the arm with plastic wrap and refrigerate for at least 1 hour, or up to 5 days.

11. Just before serving, remove the plastic wrap, then transfer the arm to a serving platter. Cut 2 slices off the back of the wrist. Serve with crudités and crackers.

12. Enjoy!

Buffalo Chicken Potato Skin Nachos

Ingredients

for 4 servings

• 4 small russet potatoes, (about 3–4 inches long and 2 inches wide), scrubbed

• 2 tablespoons canola oil, divided

• 2 teaspoons kosher salt, divided, plus more to taste

• ½ stick unsalted butter, melted

• ¼ teaspoon freshly ground black pepper, plus more to taste

• ½ cup Frank's RedHot® Buffalo Wings Sauce (120 mL)

• ⅓ cup unsalted butter (75 g)

• ½ teaspoon McCormick® cayenne pepper

• 1 ½ teaspoons distilled white vinegar

• 2 chicken breasts, boneless, skinless

• 1 teaspoon McCormick® Garlic Powder

• ½ cup chicken broth (120 mL)

• 1 ½ cups shredded mexican cheese blend (150 g), divided

Pico de Gallo

• 2 roma tomatoes

• ½ red onion, diced

• 1 jalapeño, seeded and minced

• 1 clove garlic, minced

• 3 tablespoons fresh cilantro, chopped

• ½ teaspoon kosher salt

• ¼ teaspoon ground black pepper

• lime, juiced

For Serving

• 1 cup Tasty's guacamole (260 g)

• ¼ cup blue cheese dressing (30 g)

• fresh cilantro, roughly chopped

Preparation

1. Preheat the oven to 425°F (220°C). Line a large baking sheet with parchment paper.

2. Place the potatoes on the prepared baking sheet. Pierce all over with a fork. Rub with 1 tablespoon canola oil and season with 1 teaspoon salt.

3. Bake the potatoes for 60–70 minutes, until they are soft enough to gently squeeze with an oven mitt. Remove the potatoes from the oven and let sit for 15–20 minutes, until cool enough to handle.

4. Cut the potatoes in half lengthwise and scoop out the insides, leaving a ⅛-inch-thick border of potato flesh around the edges. Cut each piece in half again lengthwise and once more crosswise to create 2-inch-long triangles.

5. Arrange the potato triangles skin-side-up in a single layer on the baking sheet and brush with the melted butter. Flip skin-side-down and brush the insides with melted butter, then season with salt and ¼ teaspoon black pepper.

6. Bake for 12–15 minutes, until the insides are golden brown. Flip the potatoes skin-side-up again and bake for 8–10 minutes more, until the skins are crispy.

7. In a medium microwave-safe bowl, combine the buffalo sauce and butter. Microwave for 30–60 seconds, until the butter is melted. Whisk well to

combine. Add the cayenne and white vinegar and whisk to combine.

8. Season the chicken breasts on both sides with 1 teaspoon salt, pepper to taste, and the garlic powder.

9. Heat the remaining tablespoon of canola oil in a large skillet over medium heat until shimmering. Add the chicken breasts and cook without moving until browned, 4–5 minutes. Flip the chicken and cook for another 3–4 minutes, until browned on the other side. Pour in the chicken broth, reduce the heat to medium-low, cover, and cook for 10–12 minutes more, or until the chicken is tender and cooked through.

10. Transfer the chicken to a medium bowl and shred with an electric hand mixer on medium-low speed, 1–2 minutes. (Alternatively, use 2 forks to

shred the chicken.) Add the buffalo sauce and ½ cup shredded Mexican cheese and mix to combine.

11. Make the pico de gallo: In a medium bowl, combine the tomatoes, onion, jalapeño, garlic, cilantro, salt, pepper, and lime juice and stir to combine.

12. Set the broiler to high.

13. Arrange the potato wedges around the edges and over the bottom of an 8-inch cast-iron skillet. Top with the buffalo chicken and sprinkle the remaining 1 cup shredded Mexican cheese on top.

14. Broil the nachos for 2–3 minutes, until the cheese is melted and bubbling.

15. Top the nachos with guacamole, the pico de gallo, blue cheese dressing, and cilantro. Serve immediately.

16. Enjoy!

Triple Chocolate Trifle

Ingredients

for 2 servings

Chocolate Pudding

• 1 cup whole milk (240 mL)

• 1 can cream

• ½ cup granulated sugar (100 g)

• ¼ cup cocoa powder (25 g)

• 3 tablespoons cornstarch

• ¼ teaspoon kosher salt

- 1 tablespoon unsalted butter, room temperature

- 1 teaspoon vanilla extract

Chocolate Whipped Cream

- 1 cup heavy whipping cream (240 mL)

- ¼ cup powdered sugar (25 g)

- 2 tablespoons unsweetened cocoa powder

Dark Chocolate Ganache

- ¼ cup heavy cream (60 mL)

- 3 tablespoons dark chocolate chip

Assembly

- 7 oz chocolate pound cake (200 g), cut into 1/2 in

- ½ cup chocolate sandwich cookie (60 g), finely crushed

• ½ cup chocolate caramel candy (100 g), chopped

• fresh raspberry, for garnish

• fresh mint leaf, for garnish

• chocolate spoon, optional, for serving

Special Equipment

• 2 wide-mouth mason jars

Preparation

1. Make the pudding: In a medium pot, combine the milk, table cream, sugar, cocoa powder, cornstarch, and salt and whisk together until evenly incorporated. Cook over medium-high heat, whisking constantly, until starting to thicken and bubble up, about 5 minutes.

2. Remove the pot from the heat and whisk in the butter and vanilla. Strain the pudding through a

fine-mesh sieve into a medium bowl. Cover with plastic wrap, pressing directly against the surface of the pudding to prevent a skin from forming. Chill in the refrigerator for at least 2 hours, or overnight.

3. Make the whipped cream: In a medium bowl, combine the heavy cream, powdered sugar, and cocoa powder. Whip with an electric hand mixer on high speed until stiff peaks form, 3–4 minutes, scraping down the sides of the bowl as needed. Transfer the whipped cream to a piping bag fitted with a large tip and chill in the refrigerator until ready to use.

4. Make the chocolate ganache: Add heavy cream to a microwave-safe liquid measuring cup. Microwave for 1 minute, until very hot. Add the chocolate chips and let sit for 2 minutes, then stir until smooth. Transfer to a piping bag fitted with a small tip. Set aside until ready to use.

5. Assemble the trifles: Transfer the chocolate pudding to a piping bag fitted with a large tip.

6. Add about ½ cup of the pound cake cubes to the bottom of each jar, pressing down to compact. Pipe about ¼ cup of chocolate pudding and ¼ cup of the whipped cream on top. Sprinkle 2–3 tablespoons of crushed chocolate sandwich cookies and 2 tablespoons chocolate caramel candy bars on top. Repeat to make a second layer with the remaining ingredients. Finish with a drizzle of chocolate ganache and garnish with fresh raspberries and a sprig of mint. Serve with chocolate spoons.

7. Enjoy!

Creamed Spinach and Parsnips

Ingredients

- 3 parsnips

- 3 tablespoons butter, divided

- 2 tablespoons honey

- 1 large bunch (or 2 medium bunches) of spinach

- 1 small onion

- 1 tablespoon olive oil

- 1 tablespoon flour

- 1 cup half and half or cream

- 1 pinch nutmeg

- Salt and pepper

Preparation

1. Clean, peel, and slice your parsnips into 1-inch batons.

2. Preheat the oven to 400° F. Par-cook the parsnips until almost cooked through in either a pot of simmering salted water for approximately 20 to 30 mins, or with a few inches of water in a slow cooker set to high heat (I cooked mine this way and it took about 3 hours).

3. When the parsnips are done, lay them in a single layer on a baking sheet and drizzle with a 2 tablespoons each of melted butter and honey.

4. Roast the parsnips in the preheated oven for 20 to 30 minutes until they start to get crispy and brown.

5. While the parsnips are roasting, clean the leaves from a large bunch of spinach and remove the tough stems. Roughly chop the spinach, blanch it in salted boiling water until bright green (less than 15 seconds), and then run it under cold water to set the color. Squeeze out the liquid and set aside.

6. Chop a small onion, and sautée it in some olive oil and butter (1 tablespoon each) on medium heat. When the onion is becoming translucent, add a tablespoon of flour and cook for another minute.

7. While the flour is cooking down, heat a cup of half and half in the microwave or on the stovetop for a minute, and then stir it slowly into the onions, whisking frequently to make sure there are no flour lumps.

8. Cook the half and half down for a few minutes until it's starting to thicken, then add a pinch of nutmeg, salt and pepper, and taste for seasoning.

9. Add your parsnips and spinach, heat through, and serve.

Booby Rolls

Ingredients

• 1 1/2 cups whole milk

• 3/4 cup unsalted butter

• 2/3 cup honey, divided

• 2 1/4 teaspoons dry active yeast (about 1 packet)

• 2 large eggs

• 1 1/2 teaspoons sea salt

• 4 1/4 cups all-purpose flour

Preparation

1. Heat milk to a simmer on the stovetop. Add 1/4 cup butter to the milk, stirring until the butter melts. Stir in 1/3 cup honey. Pour the milk into the

bowl of an electric mixer to cool a bit. When the milk mixture is barely over room temperature, sprinkle the yeast over the top. Swirl the bowl a couple times, then let the yeast sit and foam for at least 10 minutes.

2. Once the yeast looks foamy, add in the eggs and salt. Then place a bread hook on your mixer and turn the mixer on low. Slowly add the flour until the dough comes away from the sides into a ball but is still sticky. (Only add 4 1/4 cups of flour, unless extra is needed to make the dough pull away from the sides.) Once the dough pulls away from the bowl, stop the mixer; cover the bowl with a damp towel and let it rise for 1 to 2 hours, until it has doubled in size).

3. Punch the dough down and cut into 32 equal pieces with a floured knife. Then gently roll into short ropes and tie into boob knots(!!!). Place the

yeast rolls on a parchment paper lined baking sheet, about 2 inches apart, and cover with lightly dampened tea towels. Allow the rolls to rise a second time for 30 to 45 minutes.

4. Preheat the oven to 375° F. Melt the remaining 1/2 cup butter and whisk with 1/3 cup honey. Once the rolls have risen the second time, remove the towels and gently brush each roll with honey butter. Bake for 10 to 15 minutes until golden brown. Wait five minutes before serving.

Astor House Rolls

Ingredients

• 1 packet active dry yeast

• 1/2 cup lukewarm water

• 6 cups all-purpose flour, or more as needed

• 4 teaspoons kosher salt

• 1 tablespoon sugar

• 3 tablespoons unsalted butter, softened

• 2 cups whole milk, scalded and cooled to lukewarm

• 7 tablespoons plus 1 teaspoon cold unsalted butter

Preparation

1. Dissolve the yeast in the lukewarm water and let stand until foamy. Put 5 cups flour in a large bowl (you can use a mixer with a dough hook if you want) and make a well in the center. Add the yeast mixture, salt, sugar, softened butter, and milk and stir, slowly incorporating the flour from the sides. Then stir and beat the mixture until a ball of dough

has formed. Pour the dough and any remaining flour onto a work surface and gradually knead in the remaining one cup of flour.

2. Put the dough in a clean bowl, cover, and let rise until light and fluffy and almost doubled, 1 1/2 to 2 hours.

3. Punch down the dough and knead until it is smooth and elastic, about 10 minutes—you should need very little, if any, extra flour for this step. Return to the bowl, cover, and let rise until doubled in size.

4. Punch down the dough and divide into 22 pieces. Shape each piece into a tight round (Nancy Silverton instructs: cup your hand lightly around the dough, round it against the friction of a work surface to form a smooth bun, beginning slowly and increasing speed as ball becomes tighter and

smoother). Keep the other pieces covered in plastic wrap while you work.

5. Beginning with the first round, flatten each roll, seam side up, to 1/2-inch-thick. Place 1 teaspoon butter in the center, lift one edge of the dough, and pull it up and over the butter, forming a turnover-shaped roll, and pinch the edges firmly closed to seal in the butter.

6. Arrange rolls 3 inches apart on nonstick baking sheets (or baking sheets covered with parchment). Cover loosely with plastic wrap and let rise until almost doubled, about 1 hour.

7. Heat the oven to 425° F.

8. Bake until the rolls are puffed, golden, and cooked through, about 16 minutes. Cool on baking racks.

Broccoli Rabe, Potato and Rosemary Pizza

Ingredients

• Broccoli Rabe, Potato and Rosemary Pizza

• 2 uncooked pizza crusts (recipe below)

• 1 large yukon gold potato, very thinly sliced

• Salt

• Extra-virgin olive oil

• 1/2 pound broccoli rabe, washed, ends trimmed

• 1 large garlic clove, minced, plus 2 garlic cloves lightly smashed but still intact

• 1/4 teaspoon crushed red pepper flakes

• 8 ounces fresh mozzarella cheese, thinly sliced

• 2 tablespoons fresh rosemary leaves

- 1/2 cup finely grated Pecorino Romano cheese

- Freshly ground black pepper

- Rosemary sprigs for garnish

- Pizza Dough Recipe

- 2 teaspoons dry yeast

- 1/2 cup lukewarm water

- 3 1/2 cups all-purpose flour

- 1/4 cup semolina flour

- 1 teaspoon salt

- 3/4 cup cold water

- 1/4 cup olive oil

Preparation

1. Broccoli Rabe, Potato and Rosemary Pizza

2. Preheat oven to 375 F.

3. Toss potatoes with 1 tablespoon olive oil and 1 teaspoon salt in a large bowl. Arrange potatoes in one layer on a baking tray. Bake until edges begin to turn golden brown, 15 to 20 minutes. Remove from oven and let cool. Increase oven temperature to 475 F.

4. Bring a large pot of salted water to boil. Add broccoli rabe and blanch 30 seconds; drain. Plunge broccoli rabe into a bowl of ice water. Cool and drain again. Lay in one layer on a kitchen towel to thoroughly dry. Cut in 2" pieces.

5. Heat one tablespoon olive oil in skillet over medium heat. Add minced garlic and red pepper flakes. Sauté briefly, 30 seconds. Add broccoli rabe

and 1/2 teaspoon salt. Sauté one minute. Remove from heat. Taste and add more salt if necessary.

6. Assemble pizzas: Lightly brush pizza crusts with olive oil. Rub all over with smashed garlic cloves.

7. Arrange one layer mozzarella cheese over crusts. Top with one layer of potatoes and broccoli rabe. Sprinkle one tablespoon rosemary over each crust. Top with grated Pecorino cheese.

8. Bake on pizza stone or on tray on lowest rack in oven until crust is golden brown and cheese is bubbly, about 15 minutes.

9. Before serving, sprinkle with freshly ground black pepper. Garnish with fresh rosemary leaves and drizzle with extra-virgin olive oil.

1. Pizza Dough Recipe

2. Stir yeast and lukewarm water together in a bowl. Add 1/4 cup all-purpose flour and semolina. Mix well. Let sit until bubbly, about 30 minutes.

3. Combine remaining flour and salt in another bowl. Add to yeast with cold water and olive oil. Mix well to form a dough.

4. Turn dough out onto a lightly floured board and knead with hands until dough is smooth and elastic, about 10 minutes. Or use a mixer with a dough hook, and knead about 5 minutes.

5. Place dough in a lightly oiled bowl and turn to coat all sides with oil. Cover bowl loosely with plastic wrap. Let rise in a warm place until doubled in size, 1 to 2 hours. Punch dough down, and let rise another 45 minutes.

6. Divide dough into 2 equal disks (or 4 if you would like small pizzas.) Let rest 30 minutes before

shaping. Lightly flour a work surface. Using your fingers or heels of your hands, stretch the disks out to 10" shapes.

Grilled Flatbread

Ingredients

• 3 cups bread flour (396 g)

• 1 teaspoon kosher salt (3.5 g)

• 1 teaspoon instant yeast (4 g)

• 1 1/4 cups warm water (292.5 g)

• 1/4 cup extra-virgin olive oil (43 g), plus more for brushing

• Flaky salt, for finishing

• Leaves of 1 to 2 sprigs rosemary, for finishing

Preparation

1. In a large bowl, whisk the flour and salt to combine. Add the yeast and mix to combine.

2. Make a well in the center of the bowl, and add the water and olive oil. Use a wooden spoon to mix until the mixture forms a shaggy mass.

3. On a lightly floured work surface, knead the dough until it forms a smooth ball, 6 to 9 minutes (or 3 to 4 minutes on medium speed in a stand mixer fitted with the dough hook).

4. Transfer the dough to a medium, lightly oiled bowl. Loosely cover, and let rise until the dough is double in size, 30 minutes to 1 hour.

5. Preheat the grill or grill pan until smoking hot. Clean and oil the grates of the grill.

6. While the grill is heating up, divide the dough into four (roughly even) pieces; it will be on the sticky side, so oil your hands a little to make the dough easier to handle. Holding the dough on its outside edges, stretch it gently, letting gravity do most of the work to form it into an oblong shape. Lightly oil both sides of the dough. (I do this on a baking sheet that is greased in oil. I stretch the dough and place it onto the baking sheet, which is covered in oil. When I get out to the grill, I flip it over quickly to oil the other side, and, while it's still in my hand, I throw it onto the grill grates).

7. Cook until golden brown, 3 to 4 minutes per side. When the breads are still hot from the grill, brush with more olive oil, and top with flaky salt and rosemary leaves. They are best warm, but will keep for a couple days too – they make for a good picnic lunch with chicken salad, a vessel for hummus or

other dips, or . my favorite . slathered with pesto and ricotta cheese.

Pistou Bruschetta

Ingredients

• Pistou

• two bunches fresh basil

• two handfuls fresh baby spinach

• 3 cloves garlic

• lots of salt (to taste, but mine is a salty taste)

• "Soupe"

• half an onion

• 2 carrots

• half a red pepper

• one small zucchini

• 8 green beans

• 8 wax beans

• 1 roma tomato

• two ice cubes of homemade veggie stock (about 1/3 cup)

• 1 tablespoon herbes de provence

• 1 cup great northern beans

• one handful of baby spinach leaves

Preparation

1. Pistou

2. I used a mortar and pestle to make the pistou, on the advice of a well-known Mediterranean slow food chef, not to identify anyone. I found it to be a miserable, time-consuming experience and wouldn't wish it upon anyone; the basil took forever to mash, and I had to pound each little piece of garlic into submission in order to get it smaller. I ended up just chopping everything into smaller pieces anyway and then transferring them to the mortar and pestle. However, it did produce an interesting thick, pasty pistou and was enjoyable to eat. But I'm pretty sure that you could produce something pretty similar in a food processor and it would be much more efficient. To make the pistou, you combine everything together and mash it up. If you choose to use a mortar and pestle, you can try pretending that you are a rustic from the south of France and you never measure anything. Maybe that will make the process more enjoyable.

1. "Soupe"

2. I was a little more precise with my measurements in this half of the recipe because this is what I used, but you can use whatever quantities you like in yours. You can adjust the color profile easily by adding a little here or subtracting a little there. Either way, the spread is going to be beautiful! If using dry beans, soak in water overnight or for at least 3 hours before using. After soaking, rinse beans, pour into large pot and cover with water. Bring to a boil and then simmer for 30 minutes or until beans are soft, but not mushy. Drain and set aside.

3. While beans are simmering peel and chop onions and carrots into medium, but equal sized pieces. Chop red pepper, zucchini into same-sized pieces. Remove any stems from the green and wax beans

and cut on bias. Chop tomatoes into medium-sized cubes.

4. Add olive oil to large sauté pan or wok and turn to medium-high heat. Add onions and sauté for one minute. Add carrots and sauté for three minutes. Add zucchini and red peppers, and green and wax beans and sauté for 5 minutes. Then add tomato, vegetable stock, and herbes de provence. Let simmer for 10 minutes, or until carrots are tender, but not mushy. I used homemade veggie stock that I had saved in my freezer in convenient little veggie ice cubes. I strongly disadvise using store-bought veggie stock as I have found it to be mostly terrible. I used a variation of the recipe found at Veganyumyum, a popular vegan recipe blog. Here is the link: http://veganyumyum.com/2008/10/homemade-vegetable-broth/

5. Add cooked great northern beans and baby spinach leaves and cook for one more minute until these **Ingredients** are heated through. Remove from heat and spoon onto toasted Italian bread slices. Top with pistou and bit of grated parmesan or whole-milk yogurt and serve on little plates.

White Clam Pizza

Ingredients

• Homemade Pizza Dough (Makes about 20 ounces of pizza dough. Or use store-bought dough; nothing wrong with that.)

• 2 1/2 cups all-purpose flour (about 11.25 oz., or 319 grams)

• 1 1/2 teaspoons kosher or sea salt

• 3/4 teaspoon active dry yeast, or 3 grams fresh yeast (about a dime-size ball)

• 8 ounces lukewarm water (about 227 grams)

• 1/4 cup Olive oil

• For White Clam Pizza

• 24 littleneck clams, scrubbed, shucked, juices strained and reserved for another use

• 1 wedge Pecorino-Romano cheese

• 1 handful of fresh oregano, to taste

• 4 fat garlic cloves, sliced

• Good quality extra virgin olive oil

Preparation

1. Homemade Pizza Dough (Makes about 20 ounces of pizza dough. Or use store-bought dough; nothing wrong with that.)

2. These instructions are for a stand mixer, but you can do it all by hand, if you so choose. In the bowl of a stand mixer fitted with the paddle attachment, mix flour and salt together.

3. Dissolve yeast into warm water. Stir in the oil. With mixer on low speed, pour the liquid into the flour until dough comes together.

4. Scrape off the paddle and switch to the dough hook. Knead for 5 or so minutes.

5. Scrape mixer bowl and hook, and gather dough into a ball. The dough is pretty sticky, so do your best. Place in a well-oiled bowl. Cover bowl tightly with plastic wrap, lay a dish towel over it and place in a warm spot, like in the microwave. Sometimes,

before putting the dough in, I heat a mug-full of water, to get the microwave nice and warm.

6. Let rise for 1 hour. Punch dough down, and let rise for another hour.

7. This step is totally optional, but worth it if you have all day. Punch dough down again and let rise for 2 - 3 more hours. Alternatively, you can stash the dough in the fridge overnight after the first rise. Bring refrigerated dough to room temperature about an hour before forming pizzas.

1. For White Clam Pizza

2. Place a pizza stone on bottom-most rack in oven. Preheat oven to BROIL HIGH at least a half hour before you will bake the pizza.

3. Cut dough from above pizza dough recipe into two equal pieces, about 10 ounces each, weighing it with a kitchen scale if you have one. Place the

second piece of dough in a freezer bag and freeze, or make a second pizza of your choosing (e.g. dollops of ricotta cheese, a sprinkling of shredded mozzarella, and a drizzle of extra virgin olive oil on top). Yum!

4. Flatten dough very slightly, and fold in top, bottom, left side, right side, towards center. Turn over, and gently form into a round. Place on lightly floured parchment-lined sheet pan, sprinkle with flour and cover with a kitchen towel. Let rest 10 minutes.

5. Lightly oil (just a dab to keep the paper in place) a 12" pizza pan. Line with a piece of parchment paper, and lightly dust paper with flour. Place dough on paper. Dust dough lightly with flour and press down with your fingertips as you turn the pie and spread the dough evenly in all directions until you have a nice thin layer, about 1/4" thick. It

probably won't cover the entire pan; that's okay. If dough is not cooperating, it helps to let the dough rest for a few minutes.

6. Alternatively, flour your fists very well, and the ball of dough. Stretch dough over your fists and move your fists along the outside edge of the dough, stretching it out. Lay the dough on the lightly-floured parchment-lined pizza pan. Tug edges slightly to form a rough circle.

7. Scatter the clams over the dough, followed by a drizzle of olive oil, a very generous grating of Pecorino (a good half-cupful, using a microplane grater if you've got one), the oregano and the garlic. And that's it!

8. Place pan directly on pizza stone. Or, if you've got a pizza peel, pull the parchment and pizza onto the peel, then slide parchment and pizza directly onto pizza stone. Turn heat to 550 degrees F. Bake for 5

minutes, or until crust is nicely browned and crisp, and bottom of pizza has some nicely browned spots as well. Use a long-handled metal spatula or metal tongs, or the pizza peel, to lift up the pizza and take a peek underneath. 5 minutes should be plenty; don't turn your clams into rubber, please! The parchment will turn black, but it won't catch fire, so don't worry.

9. Remove from oven using the pizza peel if you have one. Cut your pizza into pieces and enjoy!

Vermont Spice Pumpkin Cake

Ingredients

• For the cake:

• 3 cups flour

- 1 teaspoon salt

- 1/4 teaspoon ground cloves

- 3/4 teaspoon nutmeg

- 2 teaspoons cinnamon

- 1 teaspoon ground ginger

- 3 teaspoons baking powder

- 1 teaspoon baking soda

- 3/4 cup butter, at room temperature

- 1 1/2 cups sugar

- 3 eggs

- 1 1/2 cups canned pumpkin

- 1/2 cup evaporated milk

- 1/4 cup water

- 2 teaspoons vanilla extract

- For the frosting:

- 3 1/2 cups sifted confectioners' sugar

- 1/3 cup butter, softened

- 11 ounces cream cheese, softened

- 2 teaspoons maple syrup

Preparation

1. cPreheat the oven to 325° F. Butter and flour two round 9-inch cake pans (I used a sheet cake pan and punched out my layers using a ring mold, hence the many layers in the photo).

2. Whisk together the flour, salt, spices, baking powder, and baking soda in a large bowl and set aside.

3. In a separate bowl or in a stand mixer, cream together the butter and sugar until light and fluffy. Add the eggs one at a time, mixing after each addition.

4. Add the pumpkin, evaporated milk, water, and vanilla, mixing after each addition.

5. Add the dry **Ingredients** and beat until just combined.

6. Pour the batter into the prepared pans and bake for 35 to 40 minutes, or until the cake springs back to the touch and pulls away from the sides of the pan. Let cool in the pans for 10 minutes, then turn the cakes out onto a cooling rack to cool fully. It's

best to chill the cakes in the refrigerators before frosting them.

7. For the frosting: Beat together all the **Ingredients** in a large bowl until smooth and fluffy.

8. If you want a cake with more layers, slice your two layers in half horizontally. Frost between each layer and top with more frosting. Leave the sides unfrosted if you like, or cover them with a thin layer of frosting.

Shrimp Asparagus Pasta

Ingredients

• 1 pound spaghetti noodles

• 2 tablespoons olive oil

• 2 garlic cloves, mined

• 1 bunch asparagus, trimmed and cut into 1 inch pieces

• 1 pound shrimp, deveined, shelled, and tails cut off

• salt and pepper to taste

Preparation

1. Cook the spaghetti noodles according to package directions. I always like a good al dente boiling.

2. While you're waiting for the noodles to cook, heat the olive oil in a large skillet under medium high heat. Add garlic and stir until fragrant, about a minute or so. Add the asparagus and cook until it softened, about 3-5 minutes. Add in the shrimp and make sure you spread them out pretty good for even cooking. Cook until the shrimp are a nice pink,

about 5-6 minutes (make sure you flip them once, in between).

3. Drain the pasta, reserving about 1 cup of liquid. Add in pasta to asparagus and shrimp mixture and pasta liquid, if needed. Season with salt and pepper to taste and serve right away!

THYROID RESET RECIPES FOR DINNER

Cottage Cheese Pancakes

Ingredients

• 1 pint fresh fruit, such as berries or sliced nectarines in summer, figs in fall (or frozen fruit anytime)

• 1/2 cup sugar

• 6 eggs, separated

• 1/2 cup whole milk

• 1 1/2 cups full-fat cottage cheese or ricotta cheese

• 1/2 cup all-purpose flour

- 1/2 teaspoon kosher salt

- 1 tablespoon sugar

- Vegetable oil for the griddle

- Crème fraîche for accompaniment

Preparation

1. In a medium pan, toss the berries and sugar over medium heat until the sugar dissolves. Set aside.

2. In a large bowl, beat the egg yolks until thick. Add the milk and beat for another 30 seconds. Gently fold in the cottage cheese.

3. In a separate bowl, sift together the flour, salt, and sugar and pour into the cheese mixture, stirring lightly.

4. With an electric mixer or whisk, beat the egg whites on medium-high speed until they are stiff

but not dry. (A helpful rule of thumb: The egg whites' stiffness should match the consistency of the **Ingredients** you fold them into; a heavy cake batter should get stiffer egg whites than a light, more liquid pancake batter.) Gently fold the whites into the batter, just until combined. It's okay if the batter is lumpy.

5. Heat a lightly oiled griddle or skillet over medium- to medium-high heat. Ladle 1/4 cup/60 ml of the batter onto the hot griddle for each pancake, leaving space between pancakes. Cook until bubbles appear on the surface of the pancakes, then flip. Hold pancakes on a rack in a low oven (200°F) until ready to serve. It's okay that the pancakes deflate on the plate. They should be lighter than air even though they present as thin, flat pancakes on the plate.

6. When done, spoon on fruit and crème fraîche and serve.

Lamb Merguez

Ingredients

• Spice Mixture - will make plenty

• 1 tablespoon coriander seed, dry toasted

• 1 tablespoon cumin seed, dry toasted

• 1 tablespoon anise seed, or fennel seed, in a pinch, dry toasted

• 1 tablespoon cinnamon, I like Ceylon

• 1/2-1 teaspoons cayenne, depending on your harissa

- 2 teaspoons turmeric

- Sausage

- 1 pound fresh ground lamb shoulder

- 2 garlic cloves, minced fine

- 1 teaspoon grated fresh ginger

- 1 tablespoon spice mix

- 2 tablespoons harissa

- 1 tablespoon tomato paste

- 1/4-1/2 teaspoons Salt, to taste

- iced water, as needed

Preparation

1. Combine the spice mix **Ingredients** and grind fine using a spice grinder or a mortar and pestle. The extra can be stored in a glass jar.

2. Using a mixer, combine all the sausage ingredients. Add the ice water, a tablespoon at a time until the mixture is well combined. If you have ground the meat yourself, you probably won't need much ice water.

3. Form a little patty and cook it off, taste and adjust the seasoning as you see fit.

4. Cover and chill this mixture overnight if you can. This will help the flavors develop. If overnight is impossible, chill at least an hour.

5. Dip your hands in ice water as you form the sausage patties. Chill the patties again if you are not going to cook them right away. Grill the merguez coils for 10-12 minutes, total, turning once.

6. I make large coils to serve four. They make a spectacular dinner party offering with lentils du puy, crusty bread, and a green salad with figs and marcona almonds.

Penne with Sweet Summer Vegetables, Pine Nuts, and Herbs

Ingredients

• 2 pints cherry tomatoes

• 2 ears corn, shucked and kernels cut off

• 2 large zucchini or summer squash, sliced in half lengthwise and then chopped into 1/2 inch thick slices

• 1 large red onion, chopped

- 2 cloves garlic, crushed

- 4 tablespoons olive oil, divided into 3 tbsp and 1 tbsp

- 8 ounces penne or farfalle pasta

- 1/3 cup torn basil leaves

- 1 tablespoon fresh oregano leaves

- Coarse salt and black pepper to taste

- 1/4 cup pine nuts (optional)

Preparation

1. Preheat oven to 450 degrees. Set a pot of boiled water on the stove to boil.

2. Toss vegetables and garlic with olive oil and season well with salt and pepper. Keep the corn separate, however. Divide all vegetables save corn

onto baking sheets and start roasting them for 35-40 minutes, or until they're vegetables are becoming sweet, golden, and slightly caramelized (to get this effect, you'll want to avoid tossing them around too much as they cook). Fifteen minutes before the end of the roasting process, add the corn, which cooks a little faster than the other vegetables!

3. If you're using the pine nuts, now is the time to toast them gently in a large frying pan set over medium heat. Stir them continually, and remove them as soon as they're becoming golden.

4. Cook pasta till tender but slightly al dente. Drain and return to pot, reserving a small amount of the cooking liquid.

5. Add the roast vegetables, along with remaining 1 tbsp olive oil and a tiny bit of the cooking liquid, to the pasta. Toss in the basil and oregano, and serve, topped with toasted pine nuts if desired.

6. Note: most fresh pastas do contain egg or milk. So use any of the popular dry brands, like Barilla or De Cecco. Whole wheat pasta if you're feeling crunchy. And if you happen to be making dinner for a vegan with a gluten allergy (or anyone with a gluten allergy), don't freak out. You can use brown rice or quinoa pasta in place of the regular pasta. They're both a fantastic option for gluten free diners, and in my opinion, much tastier and more authentic than whole wheat pasta!

Autumn Olive Medley

Ingredients

- 4 lamb shanks

- 3 tablespoons olive oil

• salt and pepper

• 2 large shallots

• 1 fennel bulb

• 1 softball-sized celery root (celeriac)

• 3 cloves garlic

• 1 bay leaf

• 1 teaspoon dried bouquet garni

• 2 cups young red wine

• 2 cups veal or beef broth

• 1 cup green olives, pits in

• 1/2 cup sundried tomatoes in oil

• 1 splash Ricard or Pernod (optional)

• finely grated zest of 1 lemon

Preparation

1. Salt and pepper the lamb shanks liberally. Heat olive oil in a large heavy pan with a tight-fitting lid. Brown the lamb shanks all over. Take your time with this and get them really nice and brown. Remove the lamb from the pan and set aside.

2. Dice the fennel bulb into small pieces. Peel the celery root and dice into the same size pieces as the fennel. Peel and chop the shallots and garlic. Lightly brown the vegetables in the pan used for the meat. When the vegetables are browned add the meat back to the pan. Add the bay leaf, the bouquet garni, the wine, and the broth. Cover the pan and simmer over medium low heat for 1 hour.

3. Add the olives and the sundried tomatoes to the pot. If necessary, add a little more wine or broth.

Simmer, covered, an additional 30 minutes, or until the meat is nearly falling off the bone.

4. If you'd like to emphasize the fennel flavor and bring out the mellowness of the olives, add a splash of Ricard or Pernod. This really does enhance the dish, and is very Mediterranean. Taste the sauce and add additional salt and/or pepper to taste. Just before serving sprinkle the lamb with the finely grated lemon zest (use a Microplane if you have one).

5. You can gently pull the meat off the bone and serve it as a stew, or as a sauce over pasta. You can also serve these on the bone as is, or over polenta. Be sure to mention to your diners that the olives contain pits!

Red Cooked Butternut Squash

Ingredients

• 1 tablespoon garlic, minced

• 2 cups beef broth

• 2 tablespoons soy sauce

• 1/2 teaspoon sesame oil

• 2 red chiles, hot ones

• 1 to 2 butternut squash, tops peeled to the orange part, no green strips they are bitter, and cut them into 1/2 inch rounds, you should have 10 to 12 rounds

• 1 teaspoon red miso paste

• sesame seeds for garnish

• scallions cut into thin rounds for garnish

• cilantro, minced for garnish

• 1 fuji apple, grated, for garnish

Preparation

1. In a sauce pan place the garlic, broth, soy sauce, sesame oil and one of the chiles. Bring the broth to a boil and then reduce the heat. This is to bring the flavors together since it is a short braise.

2. Add the squash and miso, bring it back to a boil and then reduce to a simmer and cook until it is tender. About 20 to 30 minutes.

3. Remove the squash, place in a bowl and ladle some broth over it. Place the garnishes in small bowls and let the diner choose which toppings they want. Serve.

Vanilla Date Pudding

Ingredients

• Date Pudding

• 1/2 cup brown sugar

• 3 large eggs

• 1 vanilla bean pod, seeds scraped from the inside

• 8 ounces dates, chopped

• 1 cup boiling water

• 1 teaspoon baking powder

• 1 cup all purpose flour

• 1 teaspoon white vinegar

- 1/2 teaspoon salt

- 2 tablespoons unsalted butter, melted

- Vanilla-Rum Cream

- 1/2 cup heavy whipping cream

- 2 teaspoons vanilla extract

- 1 tablespoon dark rum

- 1 tablespoon melted butter

- dash of kosher salt

Preparation

1. Date Pudding

2. Preheat your oven to 350 and butter a 9-inch pie pan.

3. Place the chopped dates in a blender. Pour over the boiling water. Let stand for 5 minutes then puree.

4. In a stand mixer, beat the eggs and brown sugar on medium high for 2 minutes. Add the vanilla seeds, vinegar, and butter and beat to combine.

5. Add a little bit of the date mixture and beat . this will bring the eggs up to temperature . add the rest and beat to combine (medium speed). Add the flour, salt, baking powder and beat just to combine.

6. Pour the mixture into your prepared pan and bake for 35 minutes or until the center is set and a cake tester comes out clean. Take a wooden skewer and poke holes every inch or so all over the pudding.

7. At this point you can let the cake cool until after dinner or pour over the vanilla-rum cream sauce

and return to the oven for 5 minutes (10 if the pudding was cooled).

1. Vanilla-Rum Cream

2. Mix the ingredients.

Savory Mushroom Bread Pudding

Ingredients

• 3 cups heaped with 1/2-inch bread cubes (about 6 ounces), I used challah

• 1 tablespoon olive oil

• 1 teaspoon butter, plus more for the baking dish

• 1 cup chopped white or yellow onion

• 1 medium garlic clove, minced

• 8 ounces Baby Bella mushrooms, or brown button mushrooms*, cut into pieces about the same size as the bread cubes

• 1 splash white vermouth, about 2 tablespoons

• 2 teaspoons chopped fresh marjoram leaves

• 2 large eggs

• 3/4 cup heavy cream, half-and-half, or whole milk

• 1/2 cup chicken or turkey stock, preferable homemade

• 3/4 cup shredded, aged, white Cheddar cheese, divided

• Kosher salt

• Freshly ground black pepper

Preparation

1. Place the cubed bread on a sheet pan and toast in a 350° F oven until somewhat dried, but not brown. Alternately, you can leave the bread out to dry overnight. It will lose some of its volume, but that's okay. Set aside.

2. Set a 10-inch skillet over medium-high heat and add the olive oil and butter to the pan. When the butter has melted add the chopped onion and a good pinch of salt. Cook until the onion begins to soften and brown a little at the edges. Add the minced garlic and stir until it is fragrant, then add the chopped mushrooms. Cook and stir until the mushrooms brown and give off some liquid. Add the vermouth and cook until the liquid reduces to a glaze. Stir in the marjoram and check the mixture for seasoning, adding more salt (if necessary) and some pepper. Remove from the heat and set aside.

3. Butter a 1 1/2-quart casserole or gratin dish. In a medium bowl, beat the eggs together with the cream and chicken stock. Add 1/2 cup of the shredded cheese and 1/2 teaspoon of salt. Taste the custard mixture and adjust the seasoning to your liking with additional salt and freshly ground black pepper. Fold the dried bread cubes and the mushroom mixture into the custard, pressing the bread down into the liquid. Let stand while you preheat the oven.

4. Preheat the oven to 350° F. Place a rack in the lower third of the oven. When the oven is heated, transfer the bread and vegetable mixture to the prepared baking dish. Press the bread down into the custard and smooth the top surface a little; sprinkle on the remaining 1/4 cup shredded cheese.

5. Place in the oven and bake for 30 to 45 minutes, or until the top is handsomely golden brown and

the custard is set. The baking time will depend on the depth of the baking dish you have chosen. Serve hot and make sure every diner gets a portion of the crusty top. Leftovers can be refrigerated, tightly covered for 2 to 3 days.

6. *If you have wild mushrooms available, you can substitute them for part of the total weight of the mushrooms.

Twice-Baked Soufflés

Ingredients

• 5 tablespoons unsalted butter

• 1/2 cup finely chopped leeks

• 1/4 cup all-purpose flour

- 1 1/2 cups whole milk, warmed

- 1 teaspoon kosher salt

- 1 pinch ground nutmeg

- 1 1/2 cups grated Parmigiano-Reggiano

- 1 cup heavy cream

- 5 eggs, separated

Preparation

1. Preheat the oven to 425°F and generously grease six 8-ounce ramekins. In a medium saucepan over medium-low heat, melt 1 tablespoon of the butter. Add the leeks and cook, stirring, until soft but not brown, 4 to 5 minutes. Transfer to a bowl and set aside.

2. Melt the remaining 4 tablespoons of butter over medium heat in the same saucepan that you used

for the leeks. When the butter stops foaming, whisk in the flour and cook, whisking, for 1 minute. Whisk in the milk and cook, whisking, until the mixture boils and thickens. Stir in the salt, nutmeg, 1 1/4 cups of the cheese, and the leeks. Transfer a third of the mixture to a bowl, whisk in the cream, and set aside. Whisk the egg yolks into the remaining two-thirds, then transfer the mixture to a large bowl.

3. In the bowl of an electric mixer fitted with a whisk attachment (or in a large bowl with a handheld mixer), beat the egg whites with a pinch of salt until they hold stiff peaks. Stir a third of the whites into the yolk mixture to lighten it, then fold in the remaining two-thirds until no streaks of white remain. Divide the mixture among the greased ramekins, smooth the tops, then run the tip of your finger around the inner edge of each ramekin (this will help the soufflé rise higher and straighter). Arrange the ramekins in a baking dish and pour

enough hot water into the baking dish to come half an inch up the side of the ramekins.

4. Transfer to the oven and bake until puffed, deep golden brown, and set within, about 25 minutes. Remove from the oven, remove the ramekins from the water bath, and let the soufflés cool (they will deflate).

5. Run a knife around the inner edge of each ramekin, then turn the soufflés out into a gratin dish and pour the reserved cream mixture over and around the soufflés. Top each with some of the reserved Parmigiano. At this point, the soufflés can be covered with plastic wrap and refrigerated for up to 24 hours (I'm telling you, this recipe is magic).

6. When you're ready to bake the soufflés a second time, preheat the oven to 425°F. Bake until the soufflés are puffed and browned (they will puff as much as—if not more than—the first time they

were baked), about 10 to 15 minutes. Serve immediately.

Orange Chiffon Cake

Ingredients

• For the orange chiffon cake:

• 2 1/4 cups cake flour

• 1 1/2 cups sugar

• 1 teaspoon baking powder

• 1 teaspoon kosher salt

• 1/2 cup canola or vegetable oil ("salad oil")

• 5 large egg yolks, at room temperature

- 3/4 cup cold water

- 1 teaspoon vanilla extract

- 1 large orange, zested

- 7 large egg whites

- 1/2 teaspoon cream of tartar

- For the Hawaiian fluff topping:

- 2 cups heavy cream

- 6 tablespoons confectioners' sugar

- 3/4 cup well-drained pineapple, diced into small pieces

- 1/2 cup dried coconut, sweetened or unsweetened

- 1/2 cup chopped, toasted, and blanched almonds

• 1/2 cup maraschino cherries, quartered [Editors'
note: we used luxardo cherries]

Preparation

1. For the orange chiffon cake:

2. Preheat the oven to 325° F. Set aside an ungreased
10-inch tube or Bundt pan.

3. In a large bowl, whisk together the flour, sugar,
baking powder, and salt. Make a well in the center
of the dry **Ingredients** and add, in order, the oil,
yolks, water, vanilla, and orange zest. Beat until
smooth.

4. In the bowl of a stand mixer fitted with the whisk
attachment, whip the egg whites and cream of
tartar on medium-high speed until very stiff peaks
form. (They should be much stiffer than for angel
food or meringue.)

5. Fold the batter gently into the egg whites.

6. Spoon the batter into the pan, smoothing the top, and bake for 50 minutes.

7. Remove the cake from the oven and immediately turn the pan upside down, sliding into onto the neck of a wine bottle or the like. Let cool completely. Once cool, use a knife or offset spatula to help loosen the cake from the side, hit the bottom of the pan sharply on a table or the counter, and remove the cake from the pan.

1. For the Hawaiian fluff topping:

2. In the bowl of a stand mixer fitted with the whisk attachment, beat the cream on medium-high speed until slightly thickened. Add in the sugar and continue to beat on medium-high until whipped to your liking. Fold in the pineapple, coconut,

almonds, and cherries. [Editors' note: We reserved some for garnish!]

3. Spoon and swirl and spread the fluff all over the cooled cake, including the inner surface.

Butternut Sage Scones

Ingredients

• 2 cups (about 9 oz. or 255 grams) all-purpose unbleached flour (I use King Arthur)

• 6 tablespoons granulated sugar, plus more for sprinkling on top of scones

• 1 tablespoon baking powder

• 1/2 teaspoon kosher salt

- 1/2 teaspoon ground cinnamon

- 1/2 teaspoon fresh ground nutmeg

- Scant ¼ teaspoon ground cloves

- Scant ¼ teaspoon ground ginger

- 2 teaspoons finely chopped fresh sage (optional)

- 6 tablespoons cold unsalted butter, cut into small cubes

- 1/2 cup butternut squash puree (see below for directions)

- 1/3 cup heavy cream, plus more for brushing on top of scones

- 1 large egg

- 8 small sage leaves

- Cinnamon drizzle, optional

Preparation

1. When measuring flour, fluff with a whisk, scoop it up with a spoon, sprinkle it into the measuring cup, and sweep off the top with the flat edge of a knife or spatula. But when I make scones, I always weigh flour, and bypass all that extra work.

2. FOR THE BUTTERNUT SQUASH: Pierce a medium butternut squash all over with a fork or tip of a knife. Place on microwave-safe dish and cook on high for about ½ hour, turning every ten minutes or so, until soft and mushy. Cut squash down the middle. If it's still hard in the middle, nuke it a little more. Scoop out seeds and pulp. Scoop out the soft squash, mash it a bit, and place in a mesh strainer over a bowl. Let drain for a couple hours, or overnight. Depending on the size of your butternut, you'll probably have extra squash, as this

recipe only uses ½ cup. Make soup with the rest. Or double the scone recipe. And make a little less soup.

3. FOR THE CINNAMON DRIZZLE: mix 1 cup confectioner's sugar with ½ teaspoon cinnamon. Add 2 tablespoons warm water. Stir until smooth. I always do this by sight, so if too loose, add more sugar. If too thick, add more water. If not cinnamon-y enough, add more cinnamon. It should be thick like corn syrup. Set aside.

4. In the bowl of a food processor fitted with the chopping blade, place the dry **Ingredients** and the chopped sage, and pulse to combine.

5. Add the butter, and pulse about 10 or so times. You want to retain some small pieces of butter. Don't blitz the heck out of it. Transfer the flour mixture to a large mixing bowl. If you've got some really large butter lumps, just squish them with the back of a fork.

6. In a large measuring cup, place the squash, egg and heavy cream. Mix well. Pour into flour mixture. With a dinner fork, fold the wet into the dry as you gradually turn the bowl. It's a folding motion you're shooting for, not a stirring motion. When dough begins to gather, use a plastic bowl scraper to gently knead the dough into a ball shape.

7. Transfer the dough ball to a floured board. Gently pat into a 6" circle. With a pastry scraper or large chef's knife, cut into 8 triangles. I use a pie marker to score the top of the dough circle and use the lines as a guide.

8. OPTIONAL BUT RECOMMENDED: Place the scones on a wax paper-lined sheet pan and freeze until solid. Once they are frozen, you can store them in a plastic freezer bag for several weeks.

9. Preheat oven to 425 degrees F. Place frozen scones on a parchment-lined sheet pan, about 1

inch apart. Brush with cream. Take the whole sage leaves, brush front and back with cream and place on tops of scones. Sprinkle tops of scones with sugar.

10. Bake for about 20 - 25 minutes, turning pan halfway through. They are done when a wooden skewer comes out clean. When cool, drizzle with cinnamon glaze.

11. Slather with clotted cream and fig jam, if you feel like gilding the lily. But if not, these are pretty darn good with just plain ol' butter, too. These are great the next day, warmed in the microwave for 15 - 20 seconds. They freeze really well, too, and can be reheated in a 350 degree F oven until warm. Enjoy!

12. BAKING TIPS: Last but not least, I highly recommend you get an oven thermometer, if you don't have one already. The success of quick breads like this depend upon a really cranking hot oven,

and if your oven fluctuates, like mine does, then you can adjust your oven temp accordingly. Mine always runs cooler, so I crank it up until the thermometer reads the temp I want. Also, if you are baking less than a full batch, double up on your baking sheets, which helps prevent scorched bottoms.

Sweet Potato Gnocchi

Ingredients

- 1 large sweet potato (about 1 pound)

- 1 cup whole-milk ricotta cheese

- 1/3 cup freshly grated Parmesan, plus more for serving

- 1 teaspoon salt

- 1 1/4 cups all-purpose flour

Preparation

1. Prick the sweet potato all over with a fork, wrap in a damp paper towel, and microwave until soft (about 7 minutes).

2. Line a baking sheet with parchment paper.

3. Scoop out the flesh of the potato and add it to a large bowl. Add the ricotta, Parmesan, and salt and mix until smooth. Add the flour, a little at a time, stirring and then kneading until the dough just comes together—don't overwork the dough as you want it stay light.

4. Once the dough comes together, divide it into 6 equal pieces. Roll each piece into a long rope, about 1" in diameter. (Dust with more flour as needed to

keep it from sticking.) Using a sharp knife, cut the rope into 1" pieces and transfer the pieces onto the parchment-lined sheet,

5. At this point, you can either freeze the gnocchi to make later (this is such a good idea for weeknight dinners!) or cook them right away. To cook, bring a large pot of salted water to a boil. Drop in the gnocchi and cook for about 2-5 minutes, or until they're tender and they float to the surface of the water. Transfer the gnocchi carefully (they're very delicate and can fall apart easily) to the parchment-lined sheet again.

6. Serve hot with more Parmesan and some cracked pepper and butter. I like to toss mine with a simple garlic sage brown butter sauce (melt butter until it smells nutty, add some sage and minced garlic and cook briefly) and sautéed greens or broccoli rabe and cheese.

Zhajiang Noodles with Eggplant

Ingredients

• For the noodles and eggplant:

• 1 pound fresh wide noodles

• 8 cups water

• 2 small eggplants

• 2 tablespoons peanut or vegetable oil, plus more as needed

• For the sauce and garnish:

• 1 tablespoon peanut or vegetable oil

• 2 tablespoons minced fresh ginger

• 8 ounces ground pork

• 1/2 medium onion, peeled and chopped into 1/2-inch pieces

• 3 cloves garlic

• 2 tablespoons mild rice wine (like Taiwan Mijiu) (See headnote)

• 6 to 8 tablespoons toasted sesame oil

• 3 tablespoons sweet wheat paste (tianmianjiang)

• 1 tablespoon soy sauce

• 2 teaspoons sugar

• 1/4 cup hot water

• 1 seedless cucumber, trimmed and julienned

• 1 green onion, trimmed and julienned (optional)

Preparation

1. Shake the noodles out onto a tea towel to loosen the strands. Cover them with a clean tea towel to keep them from drying out. In a large pot, bring the water to a boil, then turn off the heat and cover the pot to keep the water warm.

2. Clean and trim the eggplants and then cut them into 1/2-inch cubes (you should have about 1 cup) without peeling. Deep-fry or bake them in the oven: To fry them, heat the oil in a wok over medium-high and fry the eggplants until they are browned all over; to bake them, toss the eggplants in the oil and bake them at 350° F for about 15 minutes, tossing them now and then until they are completely browned. Transfer the cooked eggplant to a dish.

3. To prepare the sauce, heat the peanut oil in a wok over medium-high and add the ginger, pork, onion, and garlic. Lower the heat to medium and cook—

stirring occasionally—until the onions are translucent, about 5 minutes. Raise the heat to medium-high again and fry the mixture until the onion has browned edges, about 2 to 3 minutes.

4. Pour in the rice wine and stir it around quickly to stop the caramelization. Scoop the mixture up one side of the wok. Raise the heat to high, pour the sesame oil into the bottom of the wok and add the sweet wheat paste. Stir the paste around in the oil to break it up into a smooth layer and to fry out any raw flavors. Add the soy sauce and sugar. Mix the meat mixture into the sauce and toss the mixture around on the heat. Add the hot water and stir the sauce around to incorporate the water. Lower the heat to a simmer and let the sauce and onion mixture gently cook for 10 to 15 minutes. Add the eggplant, taste and adjust the seasoning, and cook the sauce for another 3 minutes.

5. Just before serving, bring the water to a boil and cook the noodles until done but still nice and chewy. Reserving the noodle water, use a Chinese spider or a slotted spoon to remove them to noodle bowls. Ladle the sauce on top of each mound of noodles and garnish with the cucumbers and the green onions, if using. Serve a soup bowl of the hot noodle water on the side to each person so that they may add it if they prefer a soupier base. Your diners should toss the noodles with the sauce and garnish it so that there is a nice balance of fresh, sweet, salty, chewy, and soft in each bite.

Pot Butter Chicken

Ingredients

• For the rice

- 1 cup aged basmati rice, rinsed

- 1 cup water

- 1 tablespoon ghee or vegetable oil

- 1 teaspoon salt

- For the butter chicken

- 1 (14-ounce) can diced tomatoes

- 1 tablespoon minced ginger

- 1 tablespoon minced garlic

- 1 teaspoon turmeric

- 1/2-1 teaspoons cayenne pepper (adjust to taste)

- 1 teaspoon paprika

- 1 teaspoon salt

• 2 teaspoons good-quality garam masala, divided

• 1 teaspoon ground cumin

• 1 pound boneless skinless chicken thighs, left whole

• 4 ounces butter, cut into cubes (use coconut oil, if dairy free)

• 4 ounces heavy cream (use full-fat coconut milk, if dairy free)

• 1/4-1/2 cups chopped cilantro

Preparation

1. Combine all the **Ingredients** for the rice, place in a 6 or 7-inch heat-safe pan, and set aside.

2. Place tomatoes, ginger, garlic, chicken, turmeric, cayenne, paprika, salt, 1 teaspoon of the garam masala, and cumin into the inner liner of your

Instant Pot. Mix the sauce a bit, then place the chicken. You are putting in everything except the butter, cream, cilantro, and 1 remaining teaspoon of garam masala. Mix well.

3. Place a tall steamer rack/trivet on top of the chicken mixture, and place the uncovered bowl of uncooked rice on the rack.

4. Press the Manual or Pressure cook button, set the timer to 10 mins, and cook.

5. Once it is done cooking, allow the pot to cool for 10 minutes, undisturbed. Then, release all remaining pressure and open the pot. Remove and set the cooked rice aside. Remove the chicken and set aside.

6. Using an immersion blender, blend together the sauce until it is smooth. Let the sauce cool for 5

minutes. Stir in the cut-up butter, cream, cilantro, and garam masala.

7. Remove half the sauce and freeze or refrigerate for later.

8. Break up the chicken into bite-size pieces, add it to the sauce. Serve with rice.

Beat Bobby Flay Fried Chicken Sandwich

Ingredients

• 2 chicken thighs, skinless

• 2 tablespoons flour

• 1 egg, beaten

• 4 tablespoons breadcrumbs (I used Panko)

• Salt

• Pepper

• 1+1/2 cups cider vinegar

• 1 teaspoon mustard seeds

• 1 teaspoon coriander seeds

• 2 tablespoons sugar

• 3/4 cup dill pickles, finely diced

• 1 small red pepper, grilled, peeled, seeded, and finely diced

• 1 small jalapeno, grilled, peeled, seeded, and finely diced

• 1 small white onion, finely diced

• 2 diner rolls

• 2 tablespoons mayo

• 1 handful arugula

Preparation

1. First make your relish. Bring vinegar, mustard seeds, and coriander seeds to a boil in a medium non-reactive saucepan. Cook until reduced by half and slightly syrupy. Remove from the heat, add the remaining ingredients, and gently toss to coat. Season with salt and pepper, to taste. Cover and refrigerate for at least 1 hour before serving.

2. For fried chicken heat vegetable oil in a large saucepan to 375 degrees F (190 degrees C). Season chicken with salt and pepper, coat with flour then with beaten egg and at the end toss it in Panko. Place it in the hot oil and fry until golden brown.

3. Now assemble your sandwich. Put 1 tbsp mayo on the bottom, place the arugula on mayo, then your

delicious fried chicken and top it generously with pickle relish.

Pumpkin Pavlova with Pecan Brittle

Ingredients

• For the spiced meringue and pumpkin whipped cream:

• 1/2 teaspoon ground cloves

• 1/2 teaspoon ground ginger

• 1/4 teaspoon ground nutmeg

• 2 teaspoons cinnamon, divided

• 1 cup granulated sugar

• 4 large egg whites

- 1/2 teaspoon vanilla extract

- 1 cup heavy cream

- 1 cup pumpkin purée (homemade or canned)

- 1/4 cup maple syrup

- For pecan brittle:

- 1/8 teaspoon baking soda

- 1/2 tablespoon vanilla extract

- 1 cup sugar

- 3/4 cup finely chopped pecans

- 1/4 cup shelled sunflower seeds (unsalted)

- 3 tablespoons unsalted butter, cubed

- big pinch flaky sea salt

Preparation

1. Preheat oven to 425° F.

2. On a piece of parchment paper cut to fit your baking sheet, trace two 8-inch circles in a dark marker (I use a cake pan or dinner plate). Flip the paper and place it marker-side down on your baking sheet—you'll want to be able to see the circle through to the other side.

3. In a small bowl, whisk the cloves, ginger, nutmeg, and 1 1/2 teaspoons of the cinnamon into the sugar until combined.

4. In the bowl of a stand mixer of with a handheld electric mixer, beat the egg whites until they just start to stiffen. Add spiced sugar a spoonful at a time, and then the vanilla. Continue beating until stiff peaks form.

5. Spoon the meringue into the two circles on the baking sheet. Use the back of the spoon to spread them into flat disks, about 1 1/2 inches tall (edges can be craggy). Place the baking sheet into oven and immediately turn the temperature down to 250° F.

6. After 90 minutes, turn the oven off but do not remove the baking sheet until meringues are cooled completely and have crisped up (about 1 hour). Don't open the oven door even to peek!

7. While the meringue rounds are baking and cooling, assemble the cream filling. With an electric mixer or a whisk and some elbow grease, whip the cream, pumpkin purée, remaining 1/2 teaspoon of cinnamon, and maple syrup together in a large bowl until thick and slightly thickened. Refrigerate until ready to use; you may need to give it another quick whip right before assembly.

8. To make the brittle, line a large baking sheet with aluminum foil. Set aside. In a small bowl, whisk together the baking soda and vanilla. Set aside.

9. Pour the sugar into a medium saucepan and heat over medium-high, swirling the pan around occasionally, until entirely melted into a caramelly liquid (take care not to burn it). Reduce heat to low and add the pecans, sunflower seeds, and butter. Stir until the nuts and seeds are combined and the butter is melted and incorporated.

10. Add the vanilla slurry, stirring again to combine; look alive, the mixture will froth.

11. Pour brittle mixture onto the prepared baking sheet. Spread into as thin a layer as possible, and sprinkle with sea salt. Allow to cool completely.

12. Once cool, peel the foil from the back of the brittle and break into pieces. Roughly chop large

pieces into even smaller bits, about 1/4 inch or smaller.

13. To assemble the pavlova, set one meringue round on a serving dish. Cover with a thick layer of pumpkin filling, extending to the very edges of the meringue disk. Top with second meringue layer, and then another thick spread of filling. Sprinkle with brittle bits and serve.

Mocha-Walnut Marbled Bundt Cake

Ingredients

- 2 1/4 cups all-purpose flour

- 1/2 cup finely ground walnuts

- 1 teaspoon baking powder

- 1 teaspoon salt

- 2 sticks plus 2 tablespoons (9 ounces) unsalted butter, at room temperature

- 3 ounces bittersweet chocolate, coarsely chopped

- 1/4 cup coffee, hot or cold

- 1 teaspoon finely ground instant coffee or instant espresso powder

- 1 3/4 cups sugar

- 4 large eggs

- 2 teaspoons pure vanilla extract

- 1 cup whole milk, at room temperature

Preparation

1. Center a rack in the oven and preheat the oven to 350° F. Butter a 9- to 10-inch (12-cup) Bundt pan,

dust the inside with flour and tap out the excess. (If you've got a silicone Bundt pan, there's no need to butter or flour it.) Don't place the pan on a baking sheet—you want the oven's heat to circulate through the Bundt's inner tube.

2. Whisk together the flour, ground walnuts, baking powder, and salt.

3. Set a heatproof bowl over a saucepan of gently simmering water. Put 2 tablespoons of the butter, cut into 4 pieces, into the bowl, along with the chocolate, coffee, and instant coffee. Heat the mixture, stirring often, until the butter and chocolate are melted and everything is smooth and creamy—keep the heat low so that the butter and chocolate don't separate. Remove the bowl from the heat.

4. Working with a stand mixer, preferably with a paddle attachment, or with a hand mixer in a large

bowl, beat the remaining 2 sticks butter and the sugar at medium speed for about 3 minutes—you'll have a thick paste; this won't be light and fluffy. Beat in the eggs one by one, beating well after each addition. The mixture should look smooth and satiny. Beat in the vanilla extract. Reduce the mixer speed to low and add the dry **Ingredients** and the milk alternately, adding the dry mixture in 3 portions and the milk in 2 (begin and end with the dry ingredients).

5. Scrape a little less than half the batter into the bowl with the melted chocolate and, using a rubber spatula, stir to blend thoroughly.

6. If you want to go for the gingko pattern, scrape all of the white batter into the pan and top with the chocolate. If you want a more marbled pattern, alternate spoonfuls of light and dark batter in the

pan. When all the batter is in the pan, swirl a table knife sparingly through the batters to marble them.

7. Bake for 65 to 70 minutes, or until a thin knife inserted deep into the center of the cake comes out clean. Transfer the Bundt pan to a rack and let cool for 10 minutes before unmolding, then cool the cake completely on the rack.

Green Beans & Tapenade

Ingredients

• 4 tablespoons (1/2 stick) unsalted butter

• 1 teaspoon finely minced garlic

• 1 cup heavy cream

• Kosher salt and freshly ground black pepper, to taste

• 3/4 cup finely grated Parmesan, divided

• 1 pound dried fettuccine

• 3/4 pound green beans, trimmed and cut in half crosswise (about 2-inch pieces)

• 1/2 cup Green Olive Tapenade, recipe follows, or store-bought

• 1/2 cup coarsely chopped fresh parsley

• Green Olive Tapenade

• 1 cup pitted Castelvetrano olives

• 2 anchovies, rinsed and chopped

• 1/2 teaspoon minced garlic

• 1/4 cup coarsely chopped fresh parsley

- 1/4 cup extra-virgin olive oil

- 1 tablespoon drained capers

- 2 teaspoons finely grated lemon zest

- 2 to 3 teaspoons fresh lemon juice (depending on how lemony you want it)

- Kosher salt and freshly ground black pepper, to taste

Preparation

1. In a small saucepan, melt the butter over medium heat. Add the garlic and sauté for 1 minute until it just turns golden. Whisk in the cream and bring to a simmer. Season with salt (go lightly because of the salty tapenade) and pepper, then simmer for about 8 minutes until it its reduced and thickened. Whisk in 1/2 cup of the grated Parmesan.

2. Meanwhile, bring a large pot of salted water to a boil. Cook the fettuccine according to package directions, adding the cut green beans during the last 2 minutes of cooking. Drain the pasta and green beans. Return them to the same pot, and pour in the hot Alfredo sauce. Toss to coat the pasta and beans well.

3. Immediately turn the pasta and beans into a shallow serving dish or plate it up in individual bowls. Give a final grind of black pepper, dollop over the tapenade, sprinkle over the remaining Parmesa,n and either toss yourself or let each diner toss their serving. Sprinkle with parsley as desired and serve hot.

1. Green Olive Tapenade

2. Place the olives, anchovies, garlic, parsley, olive oil, capers, lemon zest, and lemon juice in a food processor and pulse until the mixture is coarsely

blended. Taste and add salt and pepper as desired. Continue to pulse or puree until the mixture is as coarse or fine as you like. Makes: about 1 cup

Cherry-Almond Danish

Ingredients

• Basic Yeast Dough

• 3/4 cup whole milk

• 1/4 cup warm water (105° to 115° F.)

• 1 packet active dry yeast

• 1/2 cup sugar

• 1 teaspoon salt

• 2 large eggs

- 5 to 5 1/2 cups sifted all-purpose flour

- 1/2 cup unsalted butter, at room temperature

- Cherry-Almond Filling

- 2/3 cup dried cherries

- 1/4 cup rum (or other dark spirit)

- 2 egg whites

- one 7-ounce tube almond paste

- 2 tablespoons sugar

- 1/4 cup unsalted butter, at room temperature

- 1 egg yolk

- 1/4 cup sliced, blanched almonds

- Sugar, for sprinkling

Preparation

1. Basic Yeast Dough

2. The day before baking the twist: pour the milk in a small saucepan and place the pan over medium heat. When bubbles begin to form around the edges and the milk steams, remove it from the heat and let it cool to lukewarm. Measure ¼ cup lukewarm water into the bowl of a stand mixer fitted with a dough hook, or a large mixing bowl; sprinkle in the yeast; stir to dissolve.

3. Add the lukewarm milk, sugar, salt, eggs, and 1 cup flour, and blend. Mix in the butter. Beat in 2 cups of flour until the mixture is smooth. Add enough remaining flour to make a very soft dough. Knead in the mixer with the dough hook, or turn dough out onto a work surface dusted with flour and knead 3 to 4 minutes to until dough is soft and velvety and little blisters appear just under the

surface. Put into large well-greased bowl; turn dough over to bring greased side up. Cover with plastic wrap and refrigerate overnight.

4. The next day: punch the dough down (it will be quite stiff from chilling); let rise again, this time at room temperature, 60 to 90 minutes or until almost doubled. Meanwhile, proceed with the instructions for the filling.

Cherry-Almond Filling **Preparation**

1. While the dough rises, prepare the cherry almond filling: put the cherries, rum, and ¼ cup water in a small sauce pan. Bring to a simmer, cook for 2 minutes, then remove from the heat and let cool.

2. In a food processor, pulse the egg whites until foamy; crumble in the almond paste. Pulse until all the lumps are blended in. Add 2 tablespoons sugar and the butter. Set aside.

3. Heat the oven to 350 degrees, and line a baking sheet with parchment paper. Turn the dough out onto a lightly floured work surface. Cut into 2 equal pieces (4 pieces if you're making 2 twists). Roll each piece out to a 6x15-inch rectangle. Spread each rectangle with half the almond-paste mixture; dot each with half the cherries (drained of the cooking syrup). Roll each piece up from the long side, jelly-roll fashion. Pinch the edges well to seal the seam to help keep the filling inside the dough. Put the two filled rolls side by side, seams down; twist one roll over the other forming a fat rope shape. Pinch the ends of the twist to seal, and tuck under any unsightly parts!

4. Place the twist on the prepared baking sheet. Beat the egg yolk with 2 tablespoons water; brush this on top of the twist. Scatter the almonds over the twist; sprinkle with sugar. Cover; let rise until almost doubled in bulk, about 40 minutes. Bake until

browned and cooked through, 25 to 30 minutes, rotating the pan 180-degrees halfway through. Remove from the oven and transfer to a wire rack. Let cool before eating, if you have the inner strength.

Pistachio-Cherry Danish

Ingredients

• For the dough:

• 3/4 cup whole milk

• 1 vanilla bean

• 1/4 cup warm water (110° to 115°F)

• 2 1/4 teaspoons active dry yeast (one 1/4-ounce packet)

- 1/2 cup sugar

- 1 teaspoon salt

- 2 large eggs

- 5 to 5 1/2 cups sifted unbleached all-purpose flour

- 1/4 teaspoon ground cardamom

- 8 tablespoons (1 stick) unsalted butter, at room temperature

- For the filling:

- 2/3 cup dried cherries

- 1/4 cup dark rum or other dark liquor

- 2 egg whites

- 3/4 cup packed pistachio paste

- 2 tablespoons sugar

- 4 tablespoons (1/2 stick) unsalted butter, at room temperature

- Zest of 1 lemon

- 1 teaspoon unsalted butter

- 1 egg yolk, for the egg wash

- 1/4 cup coarsely chopped pistachios

- 1 teaspoon sugar, for sprinkling

- 1/8 teaspoon salt, for sprinkling

Preparation

1. Make the dough: Place the milk in a small saucepan. Split the vanilla bean in half and scrape the seeds out into the saucepan. Add the scraped, split pod to the pan, too. Warm the milk over medium heat, bringing it just under a boil. When you see little bubbles around the rim and the milk

is steaming, remove the pan from the heat and let the milk cool to lukewarm.

2. Pour the warm water into the bowl of a stand mixer fitted with the dough hook (or a large bowl); sprinkle in the yeast and stir to dissolve.

3. Add the lukewarm milk, sugar, salt, eggs, 1 cup of the flour, and the cardamom and mix together on low speed. Add the butter and mix to combine. Beat in 2 cups of the flour until the mixture is smooth. Add enough of the remaining flour to form a supersoft dough. Knead it in the mixer with the dough hook, or turn it out onto a work surface dusted with flour and knead it by hand for 3 to 4 minutes, until the dough is supple and silky smooth and small blisters develop just under its surface. Put the dough in a large well-greased bowl, turning the dough over so it's greased-side up. Cover the bowl with plastic wrap and refrigerate overnight.

4. The next day, take the dough out of the refrigerator and punch it down. Transfer it from the bowl to your countertop and cover it with a kitchen towel. Let it rise a second time, at room temperature, for up to 90 minutes, or until almost doubled in size.

5. While the dough rises, make the filling: In a small saucepan, combine the cherries, rum, and ¼ cup water. Bring the mixture to a simmer, cook it for 2 minutes, then remove it from the heat and let it cool. Drain the liquid from the mixture and set the cherries aside in a small bowl.

6. In a food processor, pulse the egg whites until they're foamy. Crumble in the pistachio paste and pulse again until it's thoroughly combined and smooth. Add the sugar and butter and pulse again to incorporate. Using a rubber spatula, scoop the

mixture into a medium bowl. Add the lemon zest and stir to combine.

7. Assemble the Danish: Preheat the oven to 350°F. Line a baking sheet with parchment paper. In a 10-inch cast-iron skillet, melt 1 teaspoon butter over low heat. Brush the melted butter over the bottom and sides of the pan to coat.

8. Turn the dough out onto a lightly floured work surface. Cut it into 4 equal pieces; you will be making 2 twists. Roll each piece out to a 5 by 12-inch rectangle. Using a rubber spatula or the back of a spoon, spread one quarter of the pistachio paste mixture on each rectangle; dot each with one-quarter of the drained cherries. Roll each piece up from the long side, jelly-roll style. Pinch the edges and ends well to seal the seams and help keep the filling inside the dough. Place 2 of the filled rolls side-by-side, seams down. Twist one roll over the

other, as tautly as possible, forming a thick rope. Pinch the ends of the twist to fuse the rolls together, and tuck or twist any less-than-pretty areas under, out of view. Repeat with the remaining rolls.

9. Coil the first twisted rope into a small, tight, snaillike spiral circle and place it in the center of the skillet. Wrap the second twisted rope around it, tucking the edges under the inner coil to connect the two ropes.

10. Beat the egg yolk with 2 tablespoons water to make an egg wash and brush the dough with it. Sprinkle the pistachios over the top, followed by the sugar and the salt. Cover the pan and let the dough rise once more until doubled in size, about 40 minutes.

11. Bake the Danish until it's browned and cooked through, 30 to 35 minutes, rotating the pan 180 degrees halfway through. Remove it from the oven,

leaving it in the skillet for a couple of minutes to set before transferring it to a wire rack to cool for about 30 minutes. You should be able to lift it out of the pan quite easily with a spatula. This is best eaten the same day it's baked. I don't even let mine cool; it's a bit messier, but I can't help myself.

Creamed Chicken a la Duchess Georgia

Ingredients

• 1 cup cooked chicken

• 1 can Cream of mushroom or other condensed cream soup

• whole milk or half and half for richness

• 1/4 cup sliced black olives

- 1/2 cup shredded monterey jack/colby cheese other preferred cheese

- 1/4 to 1/3 cups sliced white mushrooms

- 4-6 biscuits

- ground black pepper to taste

Preparation

1. Preheat oven and prep biscuits according to package instructions. If you're inclined you may make scratch biscuits instead.

2. Shred chicken in thin strips. What ever quantity you have is fine but should not be more than 1 to 1 1/2 cups or it wont be creamy enough.

3. In a double boiler, mix can of soup with milk or light cream to create sauce-like consistency in top of the boiler, cover and heat over boiling water. Do

not over dilute at this stage or it may be too runny. While soup is heating, slice black olives and small white mushrooms and shred cheese .Lightly saute mushrooms.Bake biscuits.

4. Add cheese to cream mixture, stirring until melted, then add chicken, olives, mushrooms, pepper to taste,reduce heat and simmer. If mixture is too thick add milk to desired consistency.If too thin, add more cheese.

5. Open biscuits in half on each dinner plate and cover generously with hot creamed sauce.

6. All of these **Ingredients** are added in quantities that best suit the taste of the cook and family. Since it's Monday night and I'm pooped I almost always use packaged ingredients. This recipe has infinite variations to best suit the diners and so can only be approximated.

Parisian Macarons

Ingredients

• 2 cups (200 grams) almond flour (made from blanched almonds)

• 1 2/3 cups (200 grams) confectioners' sugar

• 5 large egg whites (150 milliliters), at room temperature

• 1 drop food coloring (optional)

• 1 cup (200 grams) sugar

• 1/4 cup (60 milliliters) water

• Choice of filling: chocolate ganache, white chocolate ganache, salted caramel filling, or jam

Preparation

1. To make the macarons: If you are going to bake the macarons on baking sheets lined with parchment paper, you might want to make a template. Using a cookie cutter as your guide, trace circles about 1 1/2 inches in diameter on each sheet of paper, leaving about 2 inches between them, then turn the papers over on the baking sheets. If you're using silicone mats, there's nothing to do but line the baking sheets with them. Fit a large pastry bag with a plain 1/2-inch tip. (Alternatively, you can use a zipper-lock bag . fill the bag, seal it and snip off a corner.)

2. Place a strainer over a large bowl and press the almond flour and confectioners' sugar through the mesh. This is a tedious job, but much depends on it, so be assiduous. Then whisk to blend.

3. Put half of the egg whites in the bowl of a stand mixer fitted with the whisk attachment.

4. Add food coloring, if you're using it, to the remaining egg whites, stir and then pour the whites over the almond flour and confectioners' sugar. Using a flexible spatula, mix and mash the whites into the dry **Ingredients** until you have a homogeneous paste.

5. Bring the granulated sugar and water to a boil in a small saucepan over medium heat. If there are spatters on the sides of the pan, wash them down with a pastry brush dipped in cold water. Insert a candy thermometer and cook the syrup until it reaches 243 to 245° F. (This can take about 10 minutes.)

6. Meanwhile, beat the egg whites on medium speed until they hold medium-firm peaks. Reduce

the mixer speed to low and keep mixing until the sugar syrup comes up to temperature.

7. When the sugar syrup reaches the right temperature, take the pan off the heat and remove the thermometer. With the mixer on low speed, pour in the hot syrup, trying to pour it between the whirring whisk and the side of the bowl. You'll have spatters . it's impossible not to . but ignore them; whatever you do, don't try to incorporate them into the meringue. Raise the mixer speed to high and beat until the meringue cools to room temperature, about 10 minutes . you'll be able to tell by touching the bottom of the bowl.

8. Give the almond flour mixture another turn with the spatula, then scrape the meringue over it and fold everything together. Don't be gentle here: Use your spatula to cut through the meringue and almond mixture, bring some of the batter from the

bottom up over the top and then press it against the side of the bowl. The action is the same as the one you used to get the egg whites into the almonds and sugar: mix and mash. Keep folding and mixing and mashing until when you lift the spatula, the batter flows off it in a thick band, like lava. If you want to add more food coloring, do it now.

9. Spoon half of the batter into the pastry bag (or zipper-lock bag) and, holding the bag vertically 1 inch above one of the baking sheets, pipe out 1 1/2-inch rounds. Don't worry if you have a point in the center of each round . it will dissolve into the batter. Holding the baking sheet with both hands, raise it about 8 inches above the counter and let it fall (unnerving but necessary to de-bubble the batter and promote smooth tops). Refill the bag, pipe batter onto the second sheet and drop it onto the counter.

10. Set the baking sheets aside in a cool, dry place to allow the batter to form a crust. When you can gingerly touch the top of the macarons without having batter stick to your finger, you're ready to bake. (Depending on room temperature and humidity, this can take 15 to 30 minutes, sometimes more.) While the batter is crusting, center a rack in the oven and preheat the oven to 350° F.

11. Bake the macarons, one sheet at a time, for 6 minutes. Rotate the pan and bake for another 6 to 9 minutes, or until the macarons can be lifted from the mat or can be carefully peeled away from the paper. The bottoms will feel just a little soft. Slide the silicone mat or parchment off the baking sheet onto a counter and set aside to cool to room temperature. Repeat with the second baking sheet of macarons.

12. Peel the macarons off the silicone or parchment and match them up for sandwiching.

13. To sandwich the macarons: Line a baking sheet with parchment paper. You can use a teaspoon or a piping bag to fill the macarons. It's up to you to decide how much filling you'll want to use; some pastry chefs use enough filling to form a layer about half as high as one of the shells and others make the filling as tall as a shell, so they've got equal layers of shell, filling and shell. Spoon or pipe some filling onto the flat side of a macaron and sandwich it with its mate, gently twisting the top macaron until the filling spreads to the edges. Repeat with the remaining macarons and filling, then put the macarons on the baking sheet and cover with plastic film. (Or, if it's easier for you, pack the macs into a container.) Chill for at least 24 hours, or for up to 4 days.

14. Serving: Macarons are usually served as an afternoon treat with tea or coffee or after dinner or sometimes even after dessert. Take them out of the refrigerator about 30 minutes before serving. Storing: You must keep the macarons refrigerated for 1 day before serving, and they can stay in the fridge for up to 4 days. They can also be frozen, packed airtight, for up to 2 months; defrost, still wrapped, overnight in the refrigerator

THYROID RESET RECIPES FOR DESSERT

Dulce de Leche Dairy Dessert

Ingredients

- Dulce de Leche

- 1 (can) Sweetened Condensed Milk

- Base

- 2 cups Heavy Cream

- 1 cup Milk

- 1 (can) Dulce de Leche

- 2 teaspoons Vanilla Extract

• 1 teaspoon Sea Salt

Preparation

1. Dulce de Leche

2. Place can in either crock-pot or small pot with a lid.

3. Fill pot with water until the water level is 3/4 of the way up the can

4. Heat at lowest setting for 3-5 hours.

5. Let cool completely.

6. Try not to eat

1. Base

2. Combine all **Ingredients** until throughly blended.

3. Cover tightly and Chill for at least 2 hours (overnight preferred)

4. Put into ice cream machine and follow manufacturer's instructions.

5. When finished churning put into freezer overnight and do not touch!

6. Enjoy!

French Apple Tart (Tarte Fine aux Pommes) [vegan]

Ingredients

• 1 puff pastry

• 8.5 ounces dessert apples - for the applesauce

• 3-4 medium dessert apples

• 1 teaspoon vanilla extract

• 2 tablespoons Dairy free butter

• 2 tablespoons light brown muscovado sugar

Preparation

1. To make the applesauce, peel & core 300g [8.5oz] of apples. Place in a saucepan with 4 Tbsp of water. Cover and cook under medium heat until it has reduced to applesauce (around 10 mins). Remove from heat. Add vanilla. Leave of the side.

2. Preheat the oven to 180°C/350°F/Gas 4.

3. Roll out puff pastry to fit a rectangular oven tray. Approximatively 37 x 26cm (10 x 14.5 inches).

4. While you make the apple sauce start cutting the other apples into thin slices using a sharp knife or mandoline.

5. When the applesauce is ready, spread it evenly on top of the puff pastry leaving a thin border (2cm / 0.8 inch) all around.

6. Overlap apple slices on top to cover the whole tart.

7. Once all the apples are laid out, dot tart with dairy free butter and sprinkle sugar on top.

8. Brush some melted dairy free butter on the plain border.

9. Cook for 30mins until crisp and golden.

10. If you wish, when the tart is cooked, you can add some additional topping such as: (vegan) caramel sauce, toasted almond flakes or melted apricot jam.

Zippy Salsa Tonnato (Cold Tuna Sauce)

Ingredients

• 3 tablespoons olive oil

• 3 tablespoons unsalted butter, divided

• 1 small yellow onion, finely chopped

• 1 small fennel bulb, trimmed, cored, and diced

• 4 or 5 (1 small handful) spring radishes, trimmed and diced

• 1/2 teaspoon hot pepper flakes (or more to taste)

• 4 garlic cloves, minced

• 6 anchovy fillets

- 6- to 8- ounces can (or jar) good-quality tuna in olive oil, drained and chopped, oil reserved

- 1/2 cup dry white wine

- 1/4 cup capers, drained and rinsed

- 1/4 cup Italian parsley leaves, finely chopped, plus extra for garnish

- 1/2 cup mayonnaise or aioli

- 2 to 4 tablespoons red wine vinegar or lemon juice (start with 2 and adjust from there—I prefer more tang)

- 2 to 4 tablespoons water

- Salt and freshly ground pepper, to taste

Preparation

1. Heat the olive oil and 2 tablespoons of the butter in a skillet or saucier. Add onion, fennel, and radishes, and sauté on medium-low heat until tender and translucent. Add hot pepper flakes, garlic, and anchovies and continue sautéing over medium-low, until the anchovies have dissolved, and then stir in the tuna, mashing with the back of a wooden spoon to break up any large chunks. Raise the heat to high and add the wine. Cook until almost all evaporated, then lower the heat and stir in the capers and parsley. Swirl in the remaining 1 tablespoon of butter and remove from heat.

2. Allow to cool slightly, then transfer to a blender or food processor. Add the mayonnaise (or aioli), vinegar (or lemon juice), reserved tuna oil, and water, and process until smooth. Then let it go some more, until it is super light and airy. (You can also do this directly in the pan with an immersion blender.) Adjust for salt, pepper, acid, and—if you

prefer a little extra zip—hot pepper. You may need to add a little more olive oil or water if the purée is too thick. Serve as a dip, or tossed with pasta and a little pasta water (and something assertive and green, like arugula), or as a crostini topping, garnished with chopped parsley. [Editors' note: We spread the tonnato on a plate, then topped it with boiled potatoes, blanched asparagus and snap peas, and raw radishes and Romanesco.]

Avocado Kulfi

Ingredients

- 2 to 3 ripe avocados

- 4 tablespoons Sugar

- 1 cup coconut milk

• dairy free whipped topping (optional for garnish)

• Splash Pure Vanilla

• Pinch Ground fresh cardamom (optional)

Preparation

1. Silky smooth avocado ice cream with coconut milk, a new twist to dessert Recipe: 2 to 3 avocados 4 tbsp sugar or adjust per your taste 1 cup coconut milk to make custard like consistency (may need to add more if the avocados are too big) dairy free whip topping (optional) for garnish splash of vanilla A pinch of cardamom (optional) this will give a good Indian taste Method: Cut all the avocados and put it the a blender add sugar, vanilla, coconut milk, and cardamom blend until the mixture is a thick custard like consistency blend well and put in a freezer safe container with a lid this way it will keep away all the freezer smell. Freeze for at least 6

hours. Serve with some whipped topping Enjoy this tropical healthy non dairy ice cream all the way from the tropical Country!

Banana Cremeux

Ingredients

• 6 Ripe Bananas

• 2 cups Whole Milk

• 2 cups Heavy Cream

• 1 packet Knox Gelatin (.25oz)

• 1/2 cup Granulated Sugar

• 2 ounces Banana Liquor

• 1/2 cup White Chocolate

• 1 teaspoon Kosher Salt

• 1 Lime Zested

Preparation

1. Start by rough chopping 4 of the bananas. Set aside. Now place the milk, banana liquor, cream and sugar in a pot (thick bottom if you have one) Bring this mixture to a boil.

2. Turn off heat and add lime zest, chopped bananas, white chocolate and salt. Let this mixture steep until cool. Refrigerate overnight. (This step really helps impart the banana flavor into the dairy)

3. (Next Day) Strain the banana/dairy mixture, place into a pot and back on the stove and bring to a simmer. While it is heating up place 1 packet of gelatin into a cup with 3 Tablespoons of water.

4. Once dairy is at a simmer you can now whisk in your gelatin. Let this cook for a few minutes to dissolve all of the gelatin. Now strain the entire mixture.

5. Pour the strained Banana Cremeux base into 4oz. mason jars or into any 4oz ramekins you may have.If you fill to the top you will have enough for 8 jars. Refrigerate until set (about 6 hours) Once cold you can place the lids back on until your ready to serve.

6. Once set you can now chop the remaining bananas to place on top of the finished dessert. Optional: toast some sweetened coconut to garnish the bananas with. Enjoy!

Golden Dumplings with Whipped Coconut Cream

Ingredients

• The Dumplings

• 3/4 cup brown sugar

• 1/3 cup golden syrup

• 100 grams dairy-free butter

• 1 1/2 cups Self-Raising Flour

• 3/4 cup coconut milk

• some grated orange zest (optional)

• The whipped coconut cream!

• 1 Can of Coconut Cream (chilled)

• 2 tablespoons icing sugar

• 1 teaspoon vanilla

Preparation

1. The Dumplings

2. Combine 2 cups of water, brown sugar, golden syrup and 50g dairy-free butter in a large saucepan. Stir over a low heat until melted.

3. Meanwhile, rub together the other 50g dairy-free butter into flour with your fingertips. Add coconut milk and stir into the flour mixture until well combined.

4. Bring the sauce to the boil then drop heaped dessert spoon sized pieces of the dough into the sauce. Reduce the heat to low and simmer, covered for 15-20 minutes or until a skewer comes out clean.

Serve with the whipped coconut cream and if you want, some grated orange zest! Yum!

1. The whipped coconut cream!

2. Chill a can of coconut cream in the fridge overnight. Once opened, working fast, separate the hardened cream and liquid (keep liquid to add to a curry/milkshake or discard)

3. Still working fast, whip in icing sugar and vanilla for about 2 mins (with an electric beater or mixer)! Use immediately! Its better and thicker while still its cold!

Torta di Mele

Ingredients

- 3 1/2 apples, cored, peeled and thinly sliced

- Juice of 1 lemon

- Zest of 1 lemon

- 3 eggs

- 1/2 cup butter

- 1 cup whole milk

- 1 cup sugar

- 1 3/4 cups flour

- 1 pouch Lievito Pane degli Angeli, or substitute 1 tsp. baking powder

- *Pane degli Angeli is an Italian leavening agent lightly sweetened with vanilla. It is a common ingredient in many Italian baked goods. If you decide to buy some, search Amazon or another online gourmet foods vendor for "Lievito Pane degli Angeli."

Preparation

1. Preheat the oven to 350°.

2. Butter and flour a 9" or 10" round cake pan, preferably a springform pan. Set aside.

3. Core, peel and thinly slice the apples, and place them into a bowl. Squeeze the juice of one lemon over the apples. Stir and let rest.

4. Beat the eggs and sugar with a mixer on high speed for 5 minutes, until the mixture is light and airy.

5. Warm the butter until it is very soft but not melted and add it to the eggs and sugar, along with the milk and the zest of one lemon. Stir together.

6. If you use Pane degli Angeli, pass it through a small strainer, such as a tea strainer, to eliminate any small clumps, and add it to the batter. If you use baking powder, add it now.

7. Add the flour, and fold the dry **Ingredients** gently into into the batter, taking care not to over-stir.

8. Add the apples and mix carefully until coated.

9. Pour the batter into your buttered and floured pan.

10. Arrange slices of apple around the top surface of the cake, and bake at 350° for 50-60 minutes, until a toothpick inserted into the center comes out clean. If you wish, turn on the broiler for a few minutes at the end of cooking in order to give the top a golden brown color.

11. Serve warm or at room temperature for dessert, with afternoon coffee, or even for breakfast.

Pavlova Dessert with Fresh Summer Goodies

Ingredients

• 3 egg whites (1 egg white per layer)

• 160 grams sugar

• 1 teaspoon vanilla extract

• 1 teaspoon starch or cornflour

Preparation

1. The success of the Pavlova dessert lies in the texture of the meringue. Just for this time, you will

have to say "no" to the classic French hard meringue. If you squash Pavlova meringue lightly with your fingers, it will melt, not break. Ivory colour on the outside and white candy cotton texture inside. See below. To achieve this, you need to whip the eggs to total death and then be super patient and let the meringue cook very slowly in the oven.

2. Put together egg whites with starch, vanilla, and half of your sugar. Whip for 2-3 minutes, then add the remaining sugar. I use my favourite kitchen robot (max. speed) and the whole process takes only 4 minutes. If you are using a hand mixer, it might take unto 8 minutes. When ready, your mixture will be so thick and silky, that you can make whatever shape you want and it will not deform.

3. Now spit your mixture into three parts and put them on to the baking paper.

4. Meringue does not grow in size in really - just a bit. So, you can leave little space between the three portion. Take a table spoon and form these three parts into similar circles, creating a small groove in the middle to fit in all your berries in the end. Preheat the oven 70-90C/158-194F/fan and cook for 1.5-2 hours. If you are baking the meringue for the fir time, just keep on opening the door of the oven and checking the substance with your finger. It should be crispy on the outside, but very fragile and squashy inside. Meringue should always stay soft and moist. You should be able to lift if from the baking paper quite easily; but be carful, do not break it. It can also catch some ivory tan :). When ready, switch off the oven and keep it inside for another hour. I kept it there overnight - it does not dry easily.

5. Now take out the layers and create! Just remember: your meringue is so soft and delicate, that fruit and berries can damage it or even make it soggy; so, leave all the decorations for the last minute - right before serving. I used all fruit and berries, that I could find in my local supermarket.. some glossy powder and hard, decorative candies.

6. My Pavlova does not contain cream, because ballerinas do not eat whipped cream (even on holidays, they do not have the right to be weak). I also do not think, that this dessert needs cream. The true pleasure of the Pavlova comes from the surprisingly soft and airy meringue; while ripe, juicy fruit and berries help to cut off its bitter sweetness

Chocolate Ganache Raspberry Cream Tart

Ingredients

• 1 cup almond Meal

• 1 cup oat Flour (gluten free as needed)

• 1/4 teaspoon salt

• 3 tablespoons coconut oil

• 2 tablespoons maple syrup (the real stuff)

• 1 tablespoon water

• 1/2 teaspoon pure vanilla extract

• Chocolate Ganache (adapted from Giada's Feel Good Food – vegan chocolate truffles) and Raspberry Cream layers

• 1 cup raw unsalted cashews

• 1 cup water

• 2 cups bittersweet chocolate (dairy free/vegan if needed)

• 1 teaspoon pure vanilla extract

• 1 tablespoon maple syrup

• 1 cup raspberries (fresh or frozen)

• 1 handful fresh raspberries for topping finished tart

• 2 tablespoons raspberry jam

Preparation

1. Preheat Oven to 350 F

2. In a medium bowl combine, Almond Meal, ½ cup of the Oat Flour and salt. Next add in Coconut Oil, Maple Syrup and Vanilla. Mix completely with a fork, then add in the remaining half cup of Oat

Flour and the water. Continue to mix with a fork until the mixture resembles wet sand.

3. Lightly coat a tart shell (I use a 10 inch one with a removable bottom) with a little extra coconut oil and then pour in the crust mixture. With clean hands (you could also use a piece of wax paper or parchment), press the crust into the shell, pushing up the sides until it is even all around the sides and bottom.

4. Bake in preheated oven for 15 minutes. Note: if you wish to use the crust for a tart with a baked filling, only bake the tart for 8-10 minutes before filling and baking again. Either way, allow the tart shell to completely cool before filling.

1. Chocolate Ganache (adapted from Giada's Feel Good Food – vegan chocolate truffles) and Raspberry Cream layers

2. For the Cashew Cream: Soak 1 cup Raw Unsalted Cashews in 1 cup water for at least two hours or overnight. In a high powered blender, blend soaked Cashews and Water about 1 minute until creamy. Cashew cream will be used for the chocolate ganache, raspberry cream and as a topping.

3. For the Chocolate Ganache: In a bowl over a small pot with slightly simmering water or a double boiler, add all of the Chocolate and 2/3 cup of the Cashew Cream, stir occasionally until the chocolate is completely melted and combined with the cashew cream. Once the chocolate is melted and thoroughly mixed with the cream, remove from the heat and add in Vanilla and Maple Syrup. Allow to cool.

4. For the Raspberry Cream: In a medium saucepan over low to medium heat, add in Raspberries, Jam and 1/3 cup Cashew Cream. Stir and gently press the

raspberries to break them up until everything is melted together.

5. Finally to assemble the tart: (really the recipe comes together pretty quickly) Pour about half of the cooled chocolate ganache into the cooled tart crust. Carefully spread the ganache to completely cover the crust. Chill for about 15 minutes in the fridge. After 15 minutes, spread all of the raspberry cream over the ganache. Place in the fridge to chill again. After another 15 minutes, spread the remaining chocolate ganache over the chilled tart. I leave about ½ inch of the raspberry cream around the edges exposed without covering in ganache. Chill again in the refrigerator, this time for at least an hour to allow the ganache to fully firm up.

6. Garnish the finished tart with the remaining handful of raspberries. I like to place them all around the outer edge of the tart or you could also

arrange them all in the center, whatever you prefer. Serve with additional fresh raspberries and cream. If you don't need to keep your dessert vegan or dairy free, lightly sweetened fresh whipped cream is a perfect accompaniment. Otherwise, whip up the remaining cashew cream (you should still have about 1/3 to ½ cup left) with a bit of maple syrup and serve that alongside the finished tart. Enjoy!

Chocolate Coconut Pie

Ingredients

• For the Pie Filling

• 2 14 ounce cans Coconut Milk (full-fat)

• 5 ounces Semi-sweet Chocolate, chopped

- 1/2 cup Brown Sugar, packed

- 1 tablespoon Espresso, Vanilla Extract, Bourbon, Rum, etc. (optional, to flavor)

- For the Crust and Whipped Topping

- 1 sleeve Graham Crackers (9 sheets)

- 4 tablespoons Butter, melted

- 1 tablespoon Brown Sugar, packed

- 1 14 ounce can Coconut Milk (full-fat)

- 1 tablespoon Espresso, Vanilla Extract, Bourbon, Rum, etc. (optional, to flavor)

Preparation

1. Set up your slow cooker, and find a glass bowl that will sit steady inside the slow cooker and holds at least 6 cups (for reference, I used an 8-cup glass

Pyrex bowl). You will want there to be a couple of inches or so of room at the top of the bowl to make transferring the bowl to the slow cooker easier and less likely to spill.

2. Whisk both cans of coconut milk, brown sugar, and optional additives in glass bowl, then add in the chopped chocolate. Gently place bowl in the slow cooker, and add enough water to reach up the side of the glass bowl to the same level that the filling reaches inside the bowl.

3. Cook on the low setting for ten hours. After cooking, the filling should have thickened to about the consistency of hot pudding (for reference, my filling had cooked down about an inch). Remove glass bowl from the slow cooker (carefully!), briefly whisk the filling, then cover and place in the refrigerator for at least eight hours to thicken.

4. While the filling is cooling in the fridge, heat oven to 350 degrees Fahrenheit to make the crust. Crumble graham crackers either by hand in a Ziploc bag, or by pulsing in a food processor. Mix brown sugar into graham crackers with a fork, then mix in melted butter. Press crust into pie dish, then bake in oven for ten minutes. Allow to completely cool, at least thirty minutes.

5. Also while the filling is cooling, open chilled can of coconut milk and scrape separated solid coconut cream into chilled mixing bowl, reserving coconut water for another use. If using additional flavors, add in to coconut cream before whipping. Whip on medium speed for 3-5 minutes, until cream is thickened to the consistency of whipped cream, though it will likely be denser than standard dairy whipped cream. Store whipped cream in the refrigerator until ready to serve pie. The whipped

cream should keep its thickness in the refrigerator for at least four days.

6. Add cooled filling, which should now be a thick pudding consistency, to cooled pie crust, then refrigerate for at least an hour before serving to set.

7. Add a dollop of whipped cream on top of a slice of the pie, as it can be difficult to spread over an entire pie, then enjoy! Mondays may be tough but they can only be so terrible when they begin with pie.

Sourdough Schiacciata

Ingredients

- 520 grams all-purpose flour

- 16 grams extra-virgin olive oil

- 349 grams water

- 9 grams sea salt

- 104 grams ripe sourdough starter

Preparation

1. To the bowl of a stand mixer fitted with a dough hook attachment, and when your sourdough starter is fully fermented and ripe, add the flour, olive oil, water, salt, and starter. Mix on low speed for 1 minute until the **Ingredients** are combined. Then, increase the speed (#2 on a KitchenAid) and mix for about 5 minutes. After this time, the dough should start to cling to the dough hook, but it will still be shaggy and sticky. Transfer the dough to another bowl or container for bulk fermentation.

2. Let the dough rise, covered, for 2 hours during bulk fermentation, at warm room temperature (72 to 74°F). During this time, give the dough two sets of stretch and folds to give it additional strength, where the first set happens 30 minutes into the bulk fermentation. For each set, perform four folds, one at each direction, North, South, East, and West. For each fold, wet your hands, grab one side of the dough in the bowl and stretch it up and over to the other side. Rotate the bowl and continue folding each side. After the last fold, the dough will be neatly packaged up in the container. Cover the bowl, let it rise for another 30 minutes, give it one more set of folds, then let the dough rest for the remaining hour.

3. After two hours, your dough should have smoothed out and risen some (but not significantly) in the bulk fermentation container. If your baking pan is not non-stick, use parchment paper to line

the pan to prevent sticking. Liberally oil the interior of your baking pan with extra virgin olive oil. If using a single pan, scrape the dough out of the container directly into the prepared pan. If using two pans, gently scrape out your dough to a lightly floured work surface and divide the dough directly in half, placing one half in each pan. In either case, wet your hands and gently stretch the dough out until it resists to help it fill some of the pan, but don't worry if it doesn't fill the pan. Cover the pans to prevent a skin from forming on the dough, set a timer for 1 hour, and let the dough proof.

4. After 1 hour, uncover the pan(s), wet your hands again, and gently pick up and stretch the dough outward. Avoid pressing the dough at this point; you want to scoop up a side and extend it outward toward the rim of the pan. It's not necessary for the dough to fill the pan. Cover the pans and set a timer for 30 minutes.

5. After 30 minutes, place an oven rack in the middle of the oven with a baking stone or baking steel on top. If you don't have a baking surface, these can also be baked directly on the oven rack. Preheat the oven to 450°F or 425°F convection (which I prefer for a faster bake and a more golden crust). Set a timer for another 30 minutes to let the oven preheat and to let your dough continue to proof.

6. Now, your dough should have had a full, 2-hour proof, and your oven should be preheated. The dough should show bubbles on the surface, and it should have relaxed outward to either fill the pans or come close. The dough should look slightly risen, and if you poke it gently, it will feel light and airy. If it's still dense, give it another 15 minutes to rise and check back.

7. When the dough is ready to bake, uncover the pans. Drizzle on a good measure of extra virgin olive oil to cover, but not drench, the surface of the dough. Using wet fingers, dimple the dough assertively from top to bottom, so each dimple presses down through the dough to the bottom of the pan. Then, sparingly sprinkle on coarse sea salt to coat the top of the dough.

8. Place the pans onto your preheated baking surface in the oven and bake for 25 to 30 minutes at 450°F or 425°F convection. Rotate the pans 180° halfway through baking and keep an eye on them in the last 10 minutes to avoid overbaking—each pan and oven are different! When nicely golden-brown on top, take the pan(s) out of the oven and let the bread cool for a few minutes. Then, remove the bread from the pan(s), slice, and enjoy.

Cinnamon Swirl Whole Grain Sourdough Coffee Cake

Ingredients

- Preferment

- 330 grams whole grain flour

- 1/2 cup active starter (132g, but I don't weigh this anymore).

- 85 grams milk (any fat percentage)

- 85 grams heavy cream

- Final Cake

- 130 grams walnut pieces, toasted is ideal

- 60 grams brown sugar, light or dark

- 1 teaspoon cinnamon

• 1 teaspoon cocoa powder

• All of preferment

• 194 grams white sugar (1c)

• 1 teaspoon kosher salt (or 1/2tsp table salt)

• 1 teaspoon osmotolerant instant yeast, such as SAF Gold

• 3 large eggs, straight from fridge or at room temperature

• 2 teaspoons vanilla extract

• 10 tablespoons butter, softened

Preparation

1. Preferment

2. Mix milk and cream together. Add flour and starter to a medium bowl, and pour about 2/3 of the

dairy in (I eyeball it here). Mix until you fully hydrate the flour, or add more liquid as needed to do so. The preferment should be evenly mixed, fully hydrated, but firm and not sticky. Depending on the hydration of your starter and your flour, you may have to use a little more or less liquid than I've listed.

3. Cover and let ferment. If making cake that day, it can be at room temperature for a few hours (about 3 hours for me), until it's risen a little. Since it's so firm, it won't rise much, and should not double. If making later, cover and refrigerate for about a work day or overnight. If making the cake later, the preferment can be made the morning of, and the cake finished in the evening. You can also make the preferment the evening before you make the cake, and finish the cake the next day.

1. Final Cake

2. If you're like me and always forget to take **Ingredients** out of the fridge to warm, toast the walnuts while you're waiting to take the chill off the preferment and butter. Preheat oven to 250F, spread the walnut pieces on a baking sheet, and bake until fragrant, about 10min. Remove from heat and turn off oven. Let nuts cool. If you're on top of your mise en place, disregard this step.

3. Oil or butter a 12 cup bundt pan, set aside

4. Mix nuts, brown sugar, cinnamon and cocoa powder in a small bowl, set aside.

5. Put preferment and sugar in the bowl of a stand mixer. Sprinkle in salt and yeast. With the paddle attachment, mix on medium-low to incorporate. Mix will be dry and sandy at first, but then come together around the paddle. This should only take a minute or 2.

6. With mixer running, add eggs one at a time, letting each one mix in before adding the next. Add the vanilla with the last egg.

7. Add the butter in a few additions, letting each incorporate before adding more. This doesn't have to be very precise, 3-4 additions of butter is what I do.

8. Mix until the batter is smooth and evenly mixed, that is sufficient. Using a rubber spatula, scrape from the bottom once or twice to ensure the batter is evenly mixed. The crumb structure comes from fermentation, not from creaming the ingredients, so don't over mix. The cake batter should be smooth and scoopable (not pourable), similar to a muffin batter or maybe a little thicker.

9. Scoop about 1/3 of the batter into a prepared bundt pan and smooth it into an even layer. Sprinkle ½ of the nut spice mix on top. Scoop

another 1/3 of batter on top of the nuts, smoothing it with the spatula (and maybe your fingers) to cover the nuts. Sprinkle the rest of the nut spice mix. Scoop the rest of the batter into the pan and smooth it out. The pan should be a little over half full.

10. Cover the pan and let the batter rise until about 1 ½ inches from the top of the pan. This will vary based on how warm your space is, but in my kitchen, this normally takes about 2 ½ -3 hours.

11. Preheat the oven to 350F for about 20 minutes.

12. Bake cake, uncovered, until it reaches an internal temperature of 200F, or until a toothpick comes out with only a few crumbs if you don't have a thermometer, which is in about 45 minutes in my oven. Avoid opening the oven door for the first 30 minutes of baking. The cake does not have much oven spring, and should only rise to the top of the

pan. The visible part of the cake will get a golden color, and will form a crust (I know I said this cake is not bready, and it's not, trust me). This will soften and become tender once the cake is turned out of the pan.

13. Once the cake is done, remove from oven and let cool in the pan for 10 -15 minutes. Try not to forget about it because sugar from the nut mix could stick to the pan if it cools too much.

14. Turn the cake out of pan, and let cool completely.

15. Slice and serve for breakfast, dessert, or a quick bite with coffee or tea!

Strawberry Banana Chia Seed Pudding

Ingredients

for 4 servings

• 1 banana, mashed

• ½ cup greek yogurt (140 g)

• 1 cup almond milk (240 mL)

• 1 teaspoon vanilla extract

• ¼ cup chia seeds (40 g)

• 1 cup strawberry (150 g), diced

Toppings

• 1 banana, sliced

• 1 handful strawberry, diced

Preparation

1. Mash the banana in a medium bowl.

2. Mix the banana and the yogurt together until smooth.

3. Pour in the almond milk, vanilla extract, chia seeds, and strawberries, and mix until well combined.

4. Pour the mixture into an airtight container and refrigerate, covered for 4 hours..

5. Spoon the pudding into desired serving dish and top with sliced bananas and diced strawberries.

6. Enjoy!

Vegan Chocolate Chip Cookies

Ingredients

for 10 servings

• ½ cup sugar (100 g)

• ¾ cup dark brown sugar (165 g), packed

• 1 teaspoon salt

• ½ cup refined coconut oil (120 g), melted

• ¼ cup non-dairy milk (60 mL)

• 1 teaspoon vanilla extract

• 1 ½ cups flour (185 g)

• ½ teaspoon baking soda

• 4 oz vegan semi-sweet chocolate (115 g), chunks

• 4 oz vegan dark chocolate (115 g), chunks

Preparation

1. In a large bowl, whisk together the sugar, brown sugar, salt, and coconut oil until combined.

2. Whisk in non-dairy milk and vanilla, until all sugar has dissolved and the batter is smooth.

3. Sift in the flour and baking soda, then fold the mixture with a spatula, being careful not to overmix.

4. Fold in the chocolate chunks evenly.

5. Chill the dough for at least 30 minutes.

6. Preheat oven to 350°F (180°C).

7. Scoop the dough with an ice cream scoop onto a parchment paper-lined baking sheet. Be sure to

leave at least 2 inches of space between cookies and the edges of the pan so cookies can spread evenly.

8. Bake for 12-15 minutes, or until cookies just begin to brown.

9. Cool completely.

10. Enjoy!

Chocolate Chip Muffin Mug

Ingredients

for 1 muffin

• 1 oz chocolate chips (90 g)

• ¼ cup oat flour (20 g)

• ½ teaspoon baking powder

• 2 tablespoons honey

• 1 egg white

• ½ teaspoon vanilla extract

Preparation

1. Mix together egg white, honey, and vanilla extract in a greased coffee mug.

2. Add oat flour and baking powder and mix until combined.

3. Add in chocolate chips.

4. Microwave on high for 90 seconds (times may vary).

5. Enjoy!

Peppermint Bark

Ingredients

for 15 servings

• 25 mini candy canes

• 4 cups chocolate chips (700 g)

• ½ teaspoon peppermint extract

• 3 cups white chocolate chip (525 g)

Preparation

1. Place the mini candy canes in a zip top bag and use a rolling pin to crush them into small chunks. Transfer to a medium bowl.

2. In a separate medium bowl, stir the peppermint extract into the melted chocolate chips. Pour onto

a parchment paper-lined baking sheet and spread evenly with a spatula. Freeze for 5 minutes.

3. Take the pan out of the freezer and pour the melted white chocolate over the chocolate, spreading evenly with a spatula.

4. Sprinkle the crushed mini candy canes over the white chocolate.

5. Freeze for at least 1 hour.

6. Remove the bark from the freezer and break into pieces.

7. Enjoy!

Peanut Butter Oat Energy Balls

Ingredients

for 6 servings

• ½ cup rolled oats (40 g)

• ⅓ cup peanut butter (80 g)

• 1 tablespoon honey

• 1 tablespoon dark chocolate chip, optional

• salt, to taste

Preparation

1. Combine all **Ingredients** in a small bowl and mix until thoroughly combined.

2. Chill in the refrigerator for 30 minutes.

3. Use a spoon or tablespoon to evenly divide the mixture into 6 balls. Use your hands to form the ball.

4. Enjoy one now and save the rest for later by storing them in a sealed container in the refrigerator up to 1 week.

5. Enjoy!

Chocolate Mousse

Ingredients

for 2 servings

• 1 cup heavy cream (240 mL)

• 3 tablespoons sugar

• 2 oz chocolate (60 g), milk or dark, broken into small pieces

• ¼ cup heavy cream (60 mL), hot

- 6 raspberries, to garnish

- 2 sprigs mint, to garnish

- 2 tubes tube cookie, to garnish

Preparation

1. In a large bowl, combine the heavy cream and the sugar, beating with an electric mixer until soft peaks form when lifted from the bowl. Set aside two large spoonfuls of the whipped cream to garnish with at the end.

2. Whisk the chocolate and hot cream in a separate bowl until smooth, then fold in the mixture into the cream with a spatula until no streaks remain.

3. Split the chocolate cream mixture evenly between two martini glasses or your serving dish of choice, then chill for at least 1 hour.

4. Garnish with a spoonful of whipped cream, raspberries, mint, and the chocolate cookie.

5. Enjoy!

Red Velvet Box Cookies

Ingredients

for 24 cookies

• 1 box red velvet cake mix

• 2 eggs

• ⅓ cup vegetable oil (80 mL)

• powdered sugar, for topping

Preparation

1. Preheat the oven to 375°F (190°C).

2. Mix everything except the powdered sugar into a bowl (Batter will be thick).

3. Spoon into balls and roll in the powdered sugar.

4. Place on cookie sheets leaving about 2 inches (5 cm) between cookies. Level with a glass.

5. Bake for 8 to 10 minutes until cookies brown SLIGHTLY on the edges.

6. Enjoy!

Hummus Caesar Salad

Ingredients

for 2 servings

Hummus Caesar Dressing

• 4 tablespoons classic hummus

• 1 teaspoon whole grain mustard

• 1 teaspoon minced garlic

• 1.5 teaspoons nutritional yeast

• 1 tablespoon capers, drained and minced

• 1 tablespoon lemon juice

• 1 teaspoon white miso paste, dissolved in 1 1/2 tablespoons hot water

• 2 tablespoons extra virgin olive oil

• kosher salt, to taste

• freshly ground black pepper, to taste

Salad

• 6 cups mixed greens salad

• lemon juice, to taste

• kosher salt, to taste

• freshly ground black pepper, to taste

Preparation

1. Make the hummus Caesar dressing: In a medium bowl, combine 4 tablespoons of hummus, the mustard, garlic, nutritional yeast, capers, lemon juice, miso, and olive oil. Whisk until fully combined. Add another tablespoon of hummus if the dressing is looser than your desired consistency. Season with salt and pepper to taste. The dressing will keep in an airtight container in the refrigerator for up to 1 week.

2. Make the salad: Add the greens to a large serving bowl and lightly season with lemon juice and salt. Generously drizzle the dressing over the salad and toss to coat. Finish with more black pepper, as desired.

3. Enjoy!

Asian Chicken Chopped Salad

Ingredients

for 6 servings

• 2 chicken breasts

Marinade

• 2 tablespoons soy sauce

• 1 teaspoon sesame oil

• ½ teaspoon pepper

• ½ teaspoon red pepper flakes

• 1 garlic clove, sliced

• 1 tablespoon ginger, chopped

Dressing

- ¼ cup rice vinegar (60 mL)

- 1 tablespoon sesame oil

- 1 tablespoon soy sauce

- 1 tablespoon sugar

- 1 garlic clove, grated

- 1 teaspoon ginger, grated

Salad

- 2 romaine lettuces, chopped

- 1 cup red cabbage (100 g)

- ½ cup carrots (55 g), grated

- ¼ cup green onion (25 g), chopped

- ¼ cup cilantro (10 g), chopped

- ¼ cup almond slice (25 g)

- ¼ cup fried wonton chip (20 g)

Preparation

1. In a large bowl, combine marinade ingredients.

2. Add chicken into the bowl, coat the chicken, and marinate for 30 minutes in the fridge.

3. Fully cook chicken.

4. Cut into cubes.

5. In a mason jar, combine **Ingredients** for the dressing. Shake and set aside.

6. Prep the salad. Add all of the salad **Ingredients** into a large bowl and add the cubed chicken and dressing. Toss.

7. Enjoy!

Honey Lime Fruit

Ingredients

for 4 servings

• ½ lb fresh strawberry (225 g), quartered

• 2 kiwis, peeled and diced

• 2 mangoes, diced

• 2 bananas, sliced

• ½ lb fresh blueberry (225 g)

• 2 tablespoons honey

• 1 lime, juiced

Preparation

1. Place sliced fruits in a large bowl.

2. In a small bowl, mix honey and lime juice. Pour syrup over the fruit and mix.

3. Enjoy!

Chickpea Salad Sandwich

Ingredients

for 3 servings

• 15 oz chickpeas (425 g), drained and rinsed

• ¼ cup diced red onion (40 g)

• ½ red bell pepper, diced

• 3 tablespoons vegan mayonnaise

• ½ teaspoon dijon mustard

• ½ teaspoon garlic powder

- ½ teaspoon onion powder

- kosher salt, to taste

- freshly ground black pepper, to taste

- 1 tablespoon fresh dill, chopped

- sliced bread, for serving

- leafy green, for serving

Preparation

1. Add the chickpeas to a medium bowl and mash with potato masher until a chunky texture is reached.

2. Add the red onion, red bell pepper, vegan mayo, Dijon mustard, garlic powder, onion powder, salt, black pepper, and dill, and stir until well combined.

3. Store the chickpea salad in an airtight container in the refrigerator for up to 5 days.

4. To serve, spread the chickpea salad onto bread and top with leafy greens of choice. Wrap in parchment paper and secure with rubber band.

5. Enjoy!

Roasted Cauliflower Salad

Ingredients

for 4 servings

• 1 medium head cauliflower, cut into florets

• 3 large carrots, cut into 1-inch (2.5-cm) pieces

• 1 tablespoon ground cumin

• 2 teaspoons paprika

• kosher salt, to taste

• freshly ground black pepper, to taste

• 2 tablespoons olive oil

• ¼ medium red onion, thinly sliced

• 1 cup roughly chopped fresh Italian parsley (35 g)

Dressing

• ¼ cup tahini (60 mL)

• 1 clove garlic, grated

• 2 tablespoons lemon juice

• ¼ cup water (60 mL)

• ¼ cup olive oil (60 mL)

• kosher salt, to taste

• freshly ground black pepper, to taste

Preparation

1. Preheat the oven to 425°F (220°C). Line a baking sheet with parchment paper.

2. In a large bowl, toss the cauliflower and carrots with the cumin, paprika, salt, pepper, and olive oil until well-coated.

3. Spread the vegetables on the prepared baking sheet in a single layer and roast for 20-25 minutes, until the carrots are tender.

4. Make the dressing: In a medium bowl, whisk together the tahini, garlic, lemon juice, and water. While whisking, slowly drizzle in the olive oil until the dressing is emulsified. Season with salt and pepper.

5. In a large bowl, mix together the onion and parsley. Add the roasted cauliflower and carrots and toss well.

6. Drizzle the salad with the dressing, then serve.

7. Enjoy!

Banana Berry Fruit Salad

Ingredients

for 4 servings

• 3 bananas, sliced

• 12 oz fresh strawberry (340 g), quartered

• 12 oz fresh raspberry (340 g)

Dressing

• 3 tablespoons lime juice

• 1 tablespoon maple syrup

Preparation

1. Combine all the **Ingredients** above in a large bowl.

2. Mix the dressing **Ingredients** together and spread over fruit, mix well.

3. Enjoy!

Grilled Corn Summer Pasta Salad

Ingredients

for 6 servings

Pasta Salad

- 2 ears corn

- olive oil, for brushing

- 8 oz dried orecchiette pasta (225 g), cooked according to package instructions

- 2 cups quartered cherry tomatoes (400 g)

- ½ cup diced red onion (75 g)

- 1 avocado, diced

Cilantro-Lime Vinaigrette

- 1 ½ cups fresh cilantro (60 g)

- ⅓ cup olive oil (80 mL)

- 3 tablespoons lime juice

- 1 clove garlic, roughly chopped

- ½ teaspoon chili powder

• 2 teaspoons honey

• kosher salt, to taste

• freshly ground black pepper, to taste

Preparation

1. Microwave the corn on a microwave-safe plate on high power for 7 minutes. Remove from the microwave. Grip the corn with a dish towel, then cut off the bottom end with a serrated knife. Slide the corn out of the husk. It should come out fairly easily with none of the silky, stringy mess.

2. Brush the corn with olive oil, then place on a cast iron grill pan or outdoor grill over medium-high heat. Grill for 5-6 minutes on each side, until the kernels are slightly charred.

3. Insert the narrow end of an ear of corn into the center hole of a Bundt pan. Holding the corn steady

with one hand, saw off the kernels with the serrated knife. The kernels will fall into the pan for easy collection.

4. Make the cilantro-lime vinaigrette: Combine the cilantro, olive oil, lime juice, garlic, chili powder, honey, salt, and pepper in a food processor and blend until smooth.

5. In a large bowl, combine the pasta, corn, tomatoes, red onion, avocado, and vinaigrette and toss until evenly incorporated.

6. Enjoy!

Honey Mustard Chicken, Bacon, And Avocado Salad

Ingredients

for 4 servings

Dressing/Marinade

• 2 tablespoons olive oil

• ⅓ cup honey (110 g)

• 3 tablespoons stone ground mustard

• 2 tablespoons dijon mustard

• ½ lemon

• 1 teaspoon minced garlic

• ½ teaspoon salt

• ½ teaspoon pepper

• 4 chicken thighs, skinless and boneless

Salad

• 1 head romaine lettuce, chopped

• 1 cup cherry tomato (200 g), halved

• ¼ red onion, thinly sliced

• 1 avocado, sliced

• 1 hard-boiled egg, sliced

• ¼ cup cooked bacon (55 g), diced

Preparation

1. In a small bowl, add the olive oil, honey, stone ground mustard, Dijon mustard, lemon, garlic, salt, and pepper. Whisk until smooth.

2. Remove ½ of the marinade and refrigerate to use as a dressing.

3. Add chicken thighs to remaining marinade and let it marinate for two hours.

4. Add a teaspoon of olive oil to a nonstick pan. Sear chicken on each side until golden, crispy, and cooked through. Set aside and allow to rest.

5. Put lettuce in a large bowl, add tomatoes, red onions, avocado slices, and hard-boiled egg.

6. Slice chicken into strips and place in the salad.

7. Add the remaining marinade to the salad and toss.

8. Sprinkle bacon on top.

9. Enjoy!

Fattoush Salad

Ingredients

for 6 servings

• 2 small pita rounds

• ½ cup olive oil (120 mL), plus 2 tbs

• salt, to taste

• 2 medium hearts romaine lettuce

• 1 medium cucumber

• 2 cups cherry tomato (400 g)

• 5 scallions

• ½ cup radish (60 g), sliced

• 1 red bell pepper, seeded and diced

• 2 cups fresh parsley (80 g), chopped

• 1 cup fresh mint (40 g), chopped

• 1 ½ lemons, juiced

• 1 tablespoon white wine vinegar

• 2 cloves garlic, minced

• 2 teaspoons ground sumac, or lemon zest

• ¼ teaspoon allspice

• pepper, to taste

Preparation

1. Preheat the oven to 350°F (180°C).

2. Slice the pitas in half to make 4 thin rounds. Place the pitas on a nonstick sheet pan. Brush with 2 tablespoons of olive oil and season with salt.

3. Bake for about 5 minutes, until the outside is golden brown. Let cool until they become crispy.

4. Make 3 cuts lengthwise on each of the romaine hearts, remove the stems, and chop into smaller pieces. Rinse, drain, and add to a large salad bowl.

5. Seed the cucumber, dice it, and add it to the salad bowl.

6. Cut the tomatoes in half and add them to the salad bowl.

7. Mince the scallions and add them to the salad bowl.

8. Add the radishes, bell pepper, parsley, and mint to the salad bowl and toss to combine.

9. In a liquid measuring cup or small bowl, combine the remaining ½ cup (120 ml) of oil, the lemon juice, white wine vinegar, garlic, sumac, allspice, salt, and pepper and whisk until well-combined.

10. Pour the dressing over the salad.

11. Break the crispy pitas into small pieces and add to the salad. Toss well.

12. Enjoy!

Three Bean Salad

Ingredients

for 5 servings

• ½ red onion

• ½ large english cucumber

• ½ cup fresh parsley

• 15 oz chickpeas (425 g), 1 can, drained and rinsed

• 15 oz kidney bean (425 g), 1 can, drained and rinsed

- 15 oz cannellini bean (425 g), 1 can, drained and rinsed

- ¼ cup olive oil (60 mL)

- ¼ cup red wine vinegar (60 mL)

- ½ teaspoon dried oregano

- ½ teaspoon salt

- ¼ teaspoon pepper

Preparation

1. Thinly slice the red onion and add to a large bowl.

2. Quarter the cucumber, remove the seeds and dice, then add to the bowl with the red onion.

3. Use a fork to remove the leaves from the parsley, then finely chop and add to the bowl.

4. Add the chickpeas, kidney beans, and cannellini beans to the bowl.

5. In a liquid measuring cup or small bowl, combine the olive oil, red wine vinegar, oregano, salt, and pepper, and whisk together.

6. Pour the dressing over the salad and mix well until evenly distributed.

7. Enjoy!

Avocado And Tomato Salad

Ingredients

for 2 servings

• 1 avocado, diced

- 1 cup cherry tomato (200 g), finely chopped

- ¼ medium red onion, thinly sliced

- ½ lime, juiced

- salt, to taste

- 2 tablespoons fresh parsley, chopped

Preparation

1. Combine all **Ingredients** in a bowl and gently stir to combine.

2. Cover, and store in the refrigerator until ready to serve.

3. Enjoy!

Bacon, Lettuce, Tomato, And Avocado Salad

Ingredients

for 2 servings

• 8 strips bacon

• 1 head romaine lettuce, chopped

• 2 handfuls cherry tomato, or grape tomatoes, halved

• ½ cucumber

• 2 avocados, chopped

• 4 tablespoons olive oil

• 2 tablespoons balsamic vinegar

• 1 teaspoon mustard

• 1 teaspoon salt

• 1 lemon, juiced

Preparation

1. Cook bacon until crispy. Drain on a paper towel, then set aside.

2. Place chopped lettuce, tomatoes, cucumber, avocados and bacon in a large bowl.

3. In a small bowl, mix olive oil, balsamic vinegar, mustard, salt, and lemon juice to form the dressing.

4. Toss the salad with the dressing.

5. Enjoy!

Farro Lentil Salad

Ingredients

for 4 servings

• 3 ½ cups farro (350 g), cooked

• 1 ½ cups lentils (300 g), cooked

• 1 cup grape tomato (150 g), halved

• 1 cup cucumber (135 g), diced

• ½ cup yellow bell pepper (50 g), diced

• ½ cup red bell pepper (50 g)

• ⅓ cup fresh parsley (15 g), chopped

• ⅓ cup olive oil (80 mL)

• 2 tablespoons red wine vinegar

• 2 tablespoons lemon juice

• 1 teaspoon dijon mustard

• 1 clove garlic, minced

• 1 teaspoon italian seasoning

• ½ teaspoon salt

• ¼ teaspoon pepper

• fresh arugula, to taste, optional

Preparation

1. In a medium bowl, combine the farro, lentils, tomatoes, cucumber, yellow pepper, red pepper, and parsley.

2. In a liquid measuring cup or small bowl, combine the olive oil, red wine vinegar, lemon juice, Dijon mustard, garlic, Italian seasoning, salt, and pepper, and whisk until well-combined.

3. Pour the vinaigrette over the farro salad and toss until well-combined.

4. Distribute the farro salad into airtight containers with the arugula, if using. Refrigerate for up to 5 days.

5. Enjoy!

Sweet Potato And Chickpea Salad

Ingredients

for 4 servings

• 2 large sweet potatoes, or 3 small, scrubbed

• ½ medium red onion

• 15 oz chickpeas (425 g), 1 can, rinsed and drained

• ½ cup olive oil (120 mL)

• ¼ cup lemon juice (60 mL)

- 2 tablespoons garlic, minced

- 1 teaspoon ground cumin

- 1 teaspoon paprika

- ¼ teaspoon cinnamon

- ¼ teaspoon cayenne

- salt, to taste

- pepper, to taste

- 3 oz mixed greens (85 g)

- ¼ cup fresh parsley (10 g), chopped

- ¼ cup fresh cilantro (10 g), chopped

- dried cranberry, for garnish, optional

Preparation

1. Preheat the oven to 425ºF (220ºC).

2. Cut the sweet potatoes in small cubes and transfer on one half of a non-stick baking sheet.

3. Peel and slice the onion and set aside.

4. Add the chickpeas to the other half of the baking sheet.

5. In a liquid measuring cup with a pour spout, combine the olive oil, lemon juice, garlic, cumin, paprika, cinnamon, cayenne, salt, and pepper and mix well.

6. Pour half of the dressing over the sweet potatoes and chickpeas and mix with your hands until well-coated. Keep the chickpeas and sweet potatoes separated as much as possible.

7. Scoot the chickpeas toward the sweet potatoes and add the onions to the baking sheet. Make sure everything is spread out evenly.

8. Bake for 30 minutes, until the sweet potatoes are tender. Use tongs to stir halfway through. Let cool for 20 minutes.

9. Place the greens in a large bowl. Top with the roasted chickpeas, sweet potatoes, and onion.

10. Add the parsley, cilantro, and remaining dressing and toss to combine.

11. Top with dried cranberries, if using.

12. Enjoy!

Smashed Cucumber Salad

Ingredients

for 4 servings

• 2 medium english cucumbers

• 1 tablespoon minced red onion

• ½ teaspoon kosher salt

• 1 teaspoon sugar

• 1 teaspoon soy sauce

• 1 teaspoon rice vinegar

• ½ teaspoon sesame oil

• 1 tablespoon toasted sesame seeds

• red pepper flake, to taste

Preparation

1. Using a meat mallet or rolling pin, smash the cucumbers, then slice into bite-size pieces and transfer to a large bowl.

2. Add the red onion, salt, and sugar, and toss to combine.

3. In a small bowl, combine the soy sauce, rice vinegar, and sesame oil.

4. Drizzle the dressing over the cucumbers, then toss to coat.

5. Garnish with toasted sesame seeds and red pepper flakes.

6. Enjoy!

Steak and Avocado Salad

Ingredients

for 4 servings

• 1 lb sirloin steak (455 g), about ½ inch (1cm) thick

• salt, to taste

• pepper, to taste

• 2 tablespoons oil

• 2 hearts romaine lettuce, chopped

• 3 hard-boiled eggs, diced

• 2 avocados, diced

• 2 cups cherry tomato (400 g), halved

• 3 tablespoons caesar dressing

Preparation

1. Salt and pepper the steak on both sides, being sure to rub in the seasoning.

2. Heat the oil in a pan over high heat until slightly smoking.

3. Sear the steak for about 2 minutes per side.

4. Rest the steak on a cutting board for 10 minutes.

5. Slice the steak.

6. In a large bowl, combine the lettuce, eggs, avocados, cherry tomatoes, steak, and dressing.

7. Toss the salad until evenly coated and serve.

8. Enjoy!

Rainbow Fruit Salad With Honey Lime Dressing

Ingredients

for 4 servings

• 1 lb fresh strawberrie (455 g)

• 2 mangoes

• 4 kiwis

• 2 bananas

• 12 oz fresh blueberries (340 g)

• 2 tablespoons honey

• 1 tablespoon lime, juiced

Preparation

1. Quarter the strawberries, removing the stems and hulls, and place into a large bowl. Cut the "cheeks" off of the mangoes around the pits, dice the flesh, and scoop out of the skins into the bowl with the strawberries. Remove the ends from the kiwis and use a spoon to scoop out the flesh, then dice and add to the bowl. Slice the bananas and add to the bowl, along with the blueberries.

2. In a small bowl, mix together the honey and lime juice.

3. Pour the dressing over the fruit and mix gently until well-coated.

4. Enjoy!

Vegan Pasta Salad

Ingredients

for 4 servings

• 8 oz dried pasta (225 g), cooked

• 15 oz chickpeas (425 g), 1 can, drained and rinsed

• 1 cup broccoli floret (150 g), steamed

• ½ cup carrot (60 g), shredded

• ½ cup red onion (75 g), sliced

• ¼ cup fresh parsley (10 g)

• ¼ cup olive oil (60 mL)

• ¼ cup red wine vinegar (60 mL)

• 1 clove garlic, minced

- 1 teaspoon dried oregano

- salt, to taste

- pepper, to taste

- 1 ½ cups cherry tomatoes (300 g)

Preparation

1. In a large mixing bowl, combine pasta, chickpeas, grape tomatoes, broccoli, carrots, red onion, and parsley.

2. In a small liquid measuring cup, combine olive oil, red wine vinegar, garlic, oregano, salt, and pepper, and whisk to combine.

3. Pour dressing over pasta salad and stir until evenly distributed.

4. Transfer pasta salad into 4 containers and refrigerate for up to 5 days.

5. Enjoy!

Roasted Veggie Summer Salad

Ingredients

for 2 servings

- 2 cups carrots (240 g), sliced diagonally

- 2 cups halved baby potatoes (450 g)

- 1 cup roughly chopped yellow squash (150 g)

- 1 cup roughly chopped zucchini (150 g)

- olive oil, to taste

- kosher salt, to taste

- freshly ground black pepper, to taste

- 1 tablespoon minced fresh oregano leaves

- 3 cloves garlic, chopped

- mixed salad green

- ½ cup sliced radishes (60 g)

Chimichurri Dressing

- 1 cup fresh cilantro leaves (40 g)

- 1 cup fresh flat-leaf parsley leaves (40 g)

- 3 cloves garlic

- ½ teaspoon kosher salt

- ½ teaspoon freshly ground black pepper

- ¼ cup olive oil (60 mL)

- 1 lime, juiced

• 2 tablespoons red wine vinegar

Preparation

1. Preheat the oven to 400°F (200°C). Line a baking sheet with parchment paper.

2. Add the carrots, potatoes, yellow squash, and zucchini to the prepared baking sheet. Drizzle with olive oil and season with salt, pepper, the oregano, and garlic, then toss to evenly coat the coat the vegetables. *Note: You may need to quarter the potatoes if they are too thick so they roast faster.

3. Bake for 25-30 minutes, until the vegetables are golden brown.

4. Make the chimichurri dressing: Combine the cilantro, parsley, garlic, salt, pepper, olive oil, lime juice, and red wine vinegar in a food processor and blend until smooth.

5. Add a large handful of salad greens to a large bowl. Top with the roasted vegetables and sliced radishes.

6. Pour the chimichurri dressing over the salad and toss until evenly distributed.

7. Enjoy!

Brigadeiros

Ingredients

for 12 brigadeiros

• 2 tablespoons butter, plus more for greasing the plate

• 14 oz can of sweetened condensed milk (1 g)

• ⅓ cup cocoa powder (40 g)

• 1 cup chocolate sprinkles (170 g), for decorating

Preparation

1. In a saucepan on medium-low heat, melt the butter and add the sweetened condensed milk. Add the cocoa powder and stir continuously for 10-15 minutes, until the mixture begins to pull away from the edge of the pot; it should be very thick. It's done when you run a spoon through the center and it takes a few seconds to melt back into the center again. spread the mixture onto a buttered plate and refrigerate for 2 hours.

2. When set, butter your hands to prevent sticking, and pinch off a portion of the mixture. Roll it between our hands, until you have a ball about the size of a chocolate truffle. Repeat with the remainder of the mixture; you should have about 12

balls. Coat the brigadeiros in the chocolate sprinkles.

3. Enjoy!